Anti Inflammatory Diet

A Complete Guide for the Anti Inflammatory Diet Including 250+ proven recipes to Heal Your Immune System and Live a Healthy Life

John Carter

Anti Inflammatory Diet Cookbook

The 3 Week Action Plan – 120+ easy to follow recipes and proven meal plan to beat inflammation and for lasting body health

John Carter

Text Copyright © John Carter

Table of Content

INTRODUCTION

Toxins are integral part of our environment; they are present in air, water and simply everywhere. No matter how precautionary you are, these toxins, allergens and environmental pollutants find their way into your body. Inflammation is an auto-immune response of our body to fight-off these toxins and pollutants.

Acute and chronic are two major types of inflammation that can be triggers by hundreds of different factors. Our health can be severely affected due to both chronic and acute inflammation. Every year, millions of people fall victim to arthritis; it is a major disease caused by body inflammation. Psoriasis, ulcerative colitis, lupus, hepatitis, sinusitis, arthritis, join pain, sore throat, peptic ulcer, asthma, and flue are other major health complications triggered by body inflammation.

We can't control these allergens, toxins and pollutants, but we can control our diet. Whole foods have amazing healing power to nourish our body from within. Inflammation fighting foods are nutritionally balanced, and play a vital role to keep harmful effects of inflammation at bay.

Rising popularity of anti-inflammatory diet is self-explanatory given its health transforming abilities. The diet has been the center of attention for hundreds of health institutions and dietary clinics across the world. The anti-inflammatory nutrition can be an overwhelming area for many of you. There is nothing complex about managing body inflammation, you can easily make dietary changes without complex nutritional calculations.

Anti-inflammatory diet emphasizes on making healthy changes in your present diet. It includes healthy fruits, green vegetables, healthy cooking oils, and health fats to keep inflammation at bay. Following sections of the book provide a glance about the health benefits of the diet, best foods to eat, foods to avoid, and tips to make healthy lifestyle changes.

Explore nutrition-dense, inflammation fighting recipes in this exclusive anti-inflammatory cookbook. The recipes are packed with wholesome ingredients, and are easy to prepare at home. This book includes a 3-week diet plan along with an action plan; it greatly helps to follow the diet for a long time.

Get ready to learn making these wholesome meals and take control over inflammation. They are your secret to live a fulfilling, happy life.

A GLANCE AT AN ANTI-INFLAMMATORY DIET

WHAT IS BODY INFLAMMATION?

Inflammation is not necessarily a bad thing. As mentioned earlier, it is our body's natural reaction to external stimuli. It can be triggered by many forms of stimuli including bacteria, viruses, fungi, chemicals, allergens, environmental toxins, certain medicinal drugs, and injury to any body part. Inflammation can also be triggered by many lifestyle factors including obesity, smoking, excessive alcohol consumption, nutrient-less diet, and chronic stress.

Our immune system works in co-ordination with many other systems within our body. They form an interconnected network to complete hundreds of routine body functions. Immune system protects our body from any form of external attack; when it senses any possibility of an attach, it produces histamines and other substances to counteract it. Such histamine production often leads to pain, redness, and swelling.

Body inflammation is a strictly regulated process and it must remain under control. When it goes out of control, it starts putting our health at risk. It can be harmful and damaging to healthy tissues. That is why, inflammation should be temporary, and not permanent. Common signs of inflammation include swelling, redness, and or warming sensations around various body parts and joints. Inflammation also includes possible signs of numbness and pain.

Acute inflammation is our body's natural response to repair and heal damaged tissues. It aims at quickly cleansing our body of external stimuli. Acute inflammation is a temporary phenomenon. Chronic inflammation is not temporary; its duration varies from weeks to months. It not controlled, it can create an enormous amount of immune cells, which can lead to the development of many serious illnesses.

WHY YOU MUST CONTROL IT?

If not controlled or prevented, both acute and chronic inflammation can lead to critical health disorders to totally disrupt your lifestyle. Major critical complications include

- Carpal tunnel syndrome

- Alzheimer's disease

- Psoriasis

- Crohn's disease

- Heart attacks,

- Certain types of cancer

- Strokes

- Colitis

- Lupus

- Anemia

- Asthma

- Diabetes

- Rheumatoid arthritis

- Depression (in severe cases)

SMART TIPS FOR AN INFLAMMATION FREE LIFESTYLE

Apart from a healthy diet, you can make small, effective changes in your lifestyle to give a strong punch to inflammatory triggers. These small changes help your body to develop strong resistance against external attacks.

>> PROPER HYDRATION

The importance of water in our life is well-known. It allows us to get rid of waste products (including toxins and allergens) through kidneys. Water is a key liquid component that lubricates numerous body joints. It greatly helps to maintain an ideal health of body joints. A properly hydrated state of our body prevents the development of many inflammatory conditions. Ensure that you are keeping your body ideally hydrated by drinking plenty of water every day.

Drink at least 6-8 glasses (about 1.5 - 2 liters) of water every day to ensure optimum body hydration. Even a mild to moderate level of dehydration can cause inflammatory response or can worsen inflammation symptoms.

>> THE DIET MANAGEMENT

When you are on a mission to beat inflammation; it calls for adapting a smart dietary approach. The key is to achieve the right balance of nutrients in every day diet.

Antioxidants

Found in wholesome vegetables and fruits; they are helpful in inhibiting cell damage. They protect against inflammation and the development of Rheumatoid Arthritis.

Healthy fats

Healthy fats are essential part of any inflammation preventing diet. Healthy fats, including omega-3 fatty acids, assist to reduce inflammation. They are capable of effectively managing the symptoms of depression.

Minerals

Fresh vegetables, leafy greens, nuts, seeds etc. are high with essential minerals such as zinc, magnesium, potassium, and calcium. Processed foods and commercially packed foods lack essential minerals; they contain high amount of additives and preservatives to trigger inflammatory response. Modern-day farming practices have also contributed in the process of soil demineralization. As a result, plants are receiving less nutrition from soil.

Vitamins

Vitamins are important anti-oxidation supporters. Vitamin C helps to build collagen and repair joints. Vitamin D is known to improve bone health, and fight off inflammatory response caused by environmental allergens. Vitamin E helps to increase the production of essential cartilages in our body. Vitamin D, also referred as the "sunshine vitamin," assists to suppress the auto immune response. Moreover, it helps to control depression symptoms.

>> EXERCISE & SLEEP

Sedentary lifestyle is definitely not a great sign for anyone. If not managed in time, it can send invitations to many health complications. Mild to moderate exercise/jogging is greatly helpful to enhance the effects of anti-inflammatory diet. Even a brief 15-30 minutes of mild exercise/jogging is highly effective. You can also opt for yoga classes.

Give proper rest to your body; sleep is a great nourisher of your holistic health. Make sure that you are taking 7-8 hours of relaxing sleep every night. Hit the sack at reasonable sleeping hours. Your bedtime is also an important factor. Make a habit of switching off all electronics at least one hour before your bedtime.

In order to maintain a hassle-free meal planning, list down all the required ingredients and purchase them in one grocery store visit. Ingredients having larger pantry life can be purchased in higher quantity.

FOODS TO EAT

Anti-inflammatory diet helps to calm down our body's immune response to allergic reactions. It combats the harmful effects triggers by the exposure of toxins, allergens, bacteria, viruses, and fungi. Following are the list of inflammation fighting ingredients.

- Omega-3 fatty acids (healthy fats). They are found in eggs, wild caught fish, and grass-fed or pasture raised meat cuts.

- Nuts and seeds such as sunflower seeds, pumpkin seeds, chia seeds, almonds, walnuts, cashews, pistachio etc.

- Onions, ginger, garlic, bell peppers, pumpkin and leeks.

- Green leafy vegetables such as spinach, kale, broccoli, cauliflower, asparagus, Bok Choy etc.

- Herbs such as rosemary, basil, oregano, parsley etc.

- All types of berries, pineapple, apple, oranges, red grapes etc.

- Whole grains such as brown rice, millets, quinoa, and oats.

- Healthy oils such as coconut oil, extra-virgin olive oil, avocado oil, and sesame oil.

- Lentils, beets, avocado, green tea, coconut, mushrooms, zucchini, and beans.

- Spices such as turmeric, cinnamon, black pepper, cumin etc.

- Non-dairy milks such as almond milk, coconut milk etc.

- Red wine (In moderation).

- Honey, maple syrup, dark chocolate, and cacao powder.

FOODS TO AVOID

Following inflammation triggering foods must be avoided. Eliminate them from every day diet and clear them off your pantry shelves.

- Processes meats: They are loaded with saturated fats (sausage, hot dogs, burgers, steaks etc.)

- Unhealthy fats including lard, margarine, and shortening.

- Sugar added products (except for natural fruits): All canned products with added sugars such as soups, canned fruits, yogurts, bars etc.

- Unsweetened canned fruits, tomatoes, etc. should be consumed in moderation.

- Sugar based commercial drinks, beverages, and fruit juices.

- All processed and packaged foods: They are high with additives, artificial colors, and preservatives.

- Refined carbohydrates including white breads, white pasta, and noodles.

- Foods containing trans fats: Commercially processed foods, fried foods, candies, ice creams, and baked items (cookies, crackers, pastries, cakes, muffins etc.)

- Alcoholic beverages.

3-WEEK DIET PLAN& ACTION PLAN

Making a perfect diet plan is all about consuming breakfast and other meals with as much variety as possible. It keeps your everyday diet exciting with various flavors to enjoy. Following is a sample diet plan for 21 days (3 weeks).

Few action plans to keep in mind.

>> It is not compulsory to stick to the following meal plan. If you crave to eat any particular recipe on a given day, you can replace it. Your diet plan is perfect as long as you are including anti-inflammatory recipes.

>> For lunch, the book includes many salad and soup recipes. Lunch is a light meal and some people like to have a salad or soup. In order to keep it simple, you can choose any soup or salad recipe from the below list. That way, you will have 3 options every day to choose for lunch.

Soup and salad recipes for lunch.

- Fruit Blast Salad

- Avocado Quinoa Salad

- Pomegranate Kale Salad

- Turkey Green Salad

- Chicken Swiss Salad

- Chicken Spinach Salad

- Mushroom Lentil Soup

- Chicken Jalapeno Soup

- Broccoli Potato Soup

- Yogurt Tomato Soup

- Coconut Avocado Soup

- Spinach Mushroom Soup

>> Smoothies are complimentary to have along with morning breakfast. You can choose to have both breakfast and smoothie, or just breakfast.

>> Many people like to have just juice or smoothie as breakfast. Having just smoothie or juice for breakfast is also a perfectly healthy choice.

>> Appetizer and sides are totally optional. Some people like to have some veggies along with their meals. It totally depends on your preference.

>> Snack and desserts are also optional. Having a snack between lunch and dinner is an optional choice.

>> Desserts depend on your cravings. You can choose it to have as per your preference.

Day 1	
Breakfast	Cinnamon Banana Pancakes and/or Mint Summer Smoothie
Appetizer/Sides	Salmon Bites
Lunch	Beef Yogurt Meatballs or your choice of salad or your choice of soup
Snack	Cashew Ginger Dip
Dinner	Pork Chili Stew or Zucchini Jalapeno Pork Meal or Coconut Chili Salmon
Dessert	Quinoa Dessert Bars

Day 2	
Breakfast	Mushroom Spinach Frittata and/or Kale Pistachio Smoothie
Appetizer/Sides	Sesame Bok Choy Side
Lunch	Classic Italian Spiced Chicken or your choice of salad or your choice of soup
Snack	Zucchini Crisps
Dinner	Chicken Veggie Dinner Soup or Avocado Pineapple Pork
Dessert	Lemon Coconut Mousse

Day 3	
Breakfast	Ginger Spiced Oats and/or Fig Yogurt Smoothie
Appetizer/Sides	Baked Beet Sides
Lunch	Lamb Garlic Kebabs With Greens/Rice or your choice of salad or your choice of soup
Snack	Bean Potato Spread
Dinner	Beef Bread-Less Meatloaf or Herbed Mussels Treat
Dessert	Cherry Cobbler
Day 4	
Breakfast	Strawberry Chia Breakfast and/or Carrot Pineapple Juice
Appetizer/Sides	Spinach Stuffed Mushrooms
Lunch	Shrimp Mushroom Squash or your choice of salad or your choice of soup
Snack	Honey Bean Dip
Dinner	Tuna Potato Stew or Nutty Pork Steak
Dessert	Spiced Fruit Blast

Day 5	
Breakfast	Pepper Egg Breakfast and/or Pumpkin Cinnamon Smoothie
Appetizer/Sides	Potato Zucchini Appetizers
Lunch	Brown Rice Chicken Meal or your choice of salad or your choice of soup
Snack	Avocado Prosciutto Snack
Dinner	Brussels Chicken Meal or Black Bean Chili Potato
Dessert	Blackberry Granita

Day 6	
Breakfast	Coconut Crepes and/or Pumpkin Cinnamon Smoothie
Appetizer/Sides	Garlic Cauliflower
Lunch	Brown Rice Chicken Meal/ Salmon Broccoli Bowl or your choice of salad or your choice of soup
Snack	Evening Chicken Bites
Dinner	Orange Peas Chicken or Scrumptious Coconut Shrimps
Dessert	Apple Pear Delight

Day 7	
Breakfast	Apple Oats Granola and/or Avocado Cocoa Smoothie
Appetizer/Sides	Lentil Potato Patties
Lunch	Chickpea Lettuce Wraps or your choice of salad or your choice of soup
Snack	Buckwheat Evening Delight
Dinner	Garlic Basil Pork Chops or Fish Shrimp Soup
Dessert	Pumpkin Pecan Treat

Day 8	
Breakfast	Classic Banana Almond Pancakes and/or Fig Yogurt Smoothie
Appetizer/Sides	Potato Zucchini Appetizers
Lunch	Cinnamon Pork Chops or your choice of salad or your choice of soup
Snack	Evening Chicken Bites
Dinner	Couscous Carrot Chicken or Kale Cod Secret
Dessert	Lemon Coconut Mousse

Day 9	
Breakfast	Quinoa Blueberry Bowl and/or Mint Summer Smoothie
Appetizer/Sides	Spinach Stuffed Mushrooms
Lunch	Turkey Lunch Wraps/Cups or your choice of salad or your choice of soup
Snack	Avocado Prosciutto Snack
Dinner	Berry Chops Dinner or Herbed Tomato Chops
Dessert	Quinoa Dessert Bars

Day 10	
Breakfast	Cheddar Spinach Frittata and/or Kale Pistachio Smoothie
Appetizer/Sides	Baked Beet Sides
Lunch	Spinach Sea Bass Lunch or your choice of salad or your choice of soup
Snack	Zucchini Crisps
Dinner	Artichoke Chicken Stew or Chickpea Raisin Curry
Dessert	Apple Pear Delight

Day 11	
Breakfast	Ginger Spiced Oats and/or Turmeric Cinnamon Hot Milk
Appetizer/Sides	Sesame Bok Choy Side
Lunch	Oregano Lettuce Shrimp/ Mexican Pepper Salmon or your choice of salad or your choice of soup
Snack	Bean Potato Spread
Dinner	Spinach Baked Chicken or Honey Scallops
Dessert	Pumpkin Pecan Treat

Day 12	
Breakfast	Cinnamon Banana Pancakes and/or Kale Pistachio Smoothie
Appetizer/Sides	Garlic Cauliflower
Lunch	Mushroom Rice Bowl or your choice of salad or your choice of soup
Snack	Honey Bean Dip
Dinner	Fish Shrimp Soup or Bean Chicken Chili
Dessert	Blackberry Granita

Day 13	
Breakfast	Mushroom Spinach Frittata and/or Carrot Pineapple Juice
Appetizer/Sides	Salmon Bites
Lunch	Mustard Lamb Lunch or your choice of salad or your choice of soup
Snack	Zucchini Crisps
Dinner	Shrimp Scallops Stew or Cauliflower Lamb Meal or Avocado Pineapple Pork
Dessert	Spiced Fruit Blast

Day 14	
Breakfast	Hemp Chia Porridge and/or Kale Pistachio Smoothie
Appetizer/Sides	Lentil Potato Patties
Lunch	Garlic Cod Meal or your choice of salad or your choice of soup
Snack	Bean Potato Spread
Dinner	Sweet Potato Whole Chicken or Beet Haddock Dinner
Dessert	Cherry Cobbler

Day 15	
Breakfast	Pepper Egg Breakfast and/or Mint Summer Smoothie
Appetizer/Sides	Garlic Tomato Sides
Lunch	Cauliflower Coconut Curry or your choice of salad or your choice of soup
Snack	Cashew Ginger Dip
Dinner	Brussels Chicken Meal OrZucchini Buckwheat Pasta
Dessert	Lemon Coconut Mousse

Day 16	
Breakfast	Strawberry Chia Breakfast and/or Turmeric Cinnamon Hot Milk
Appetizer/Sides	Awesome Asparagus
Lunch	Broccoli Chicken Light Casserole or your choice of salad or your choice of soup
Snack	Buckwheat Evening Delight
Dinner	Sprouts Pork Soup or Grilled Mint Chops or Apple Pork Raisins
Dessert	Quinoa Dessert Bars

Day 17	
Breakfast	Coconut Crepes and/or Fig Yogurt Smoothie
Appetizer/Sides	Garlic Kale Sides
Lunch	Cod Cucumber Delight or your choice of salad or your choice of soup
Snack	Spiced Chickpeas
Dinner	Bean Chicken Chili or Bok Choy Steak Dinner
Dessert	Apple Pear Delight

Day 18	
Breakfast	Apple Oats Granola and/or Avocado Cocoa Smoothie
Appetizer/Sides	Potato Zucchini Appetizers
Lunch	Chickpea Patties or your choice of salad or your choice of soup
Snack	Evening Chicken Bites
Dinner	Herbed Broccoli Chicken or Fennel Baked Cod
Dessert	Pumpkin Pecan Treat

Day 19	
Breakfast	Classic Banana Almond Pancakes and/or Pumpkin Cinnamon Smoothie
Appetizer/Sides	Spinach Stuffed Mushrooms
Lunch	Cinnamon Pork Chops or your choice of salad or your choice of soup
Snack	Avocado Prosciutto Snack
Dinner	Chicken White Bean Soup or Stuffed Pepper Delight
Dessert	Blackberry Granita

Day 20	
Breakfast	Classic Banana Almond Pancakes and/or Cherry Beet Smoothie
Appetizer/Sides	Baked Beet Sides
Lunch	Salmon Greens or your choice of salad or your choice of soup
Snack	Honey Bean Dip
Dinner	Sprouts Pork Chops or Brown Rice Lentils
Dessert	Spiced Fruit Blast

Day 21	
Breakfast	Quinoa Blueberry Bowl and/or Pineapple Lush Red Smoothie
Appetizer/Sides	Sesame Bok Choy Side
Lunch	Chickpea Veggie Lunch or your choice of salad or your choice of soup
Snack	Zucchini Crisps
Dinner	Eggplant Pork Stew or Orange Peas Chicken or Fish Curry Dinner
Dessert	Cherry Cobbler

Breakfast
&
Smoothies

Mushroom Spinach Frittata

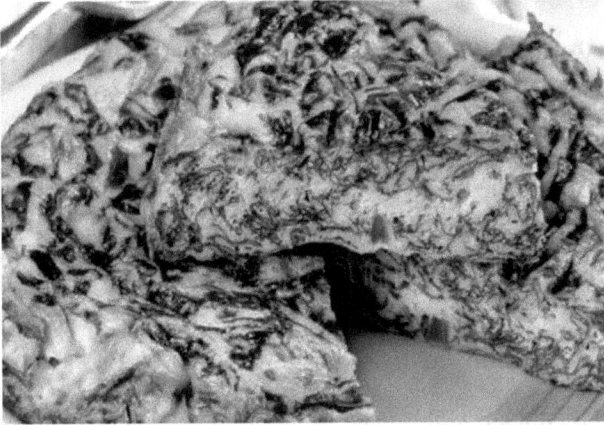

Recipe Time: 25 minutes

Serving Size: 4

Diet Type: Gluten Free, Soy Free, Dairy Free, Nut Free

Ingredients:

- 2 tablespoons avocado or coconut oil
- 8 eggs
- 2 leeks, finely chopped
- ½ teaspoon garlic powder
- ½ teaspoon dried basil
- 1 cup cremini mushrooms, (cut into slices)
- 1 cup baby spinach leaves
- Ground black pepper to taste
- ¾ teaspoon salt

Cooking Instructions:

1. Preheat an oven to 400°F.

2. Take an ovenproof skillet or saucepan (large size). In the skillet or saucepan, heat the oil over medium-high flame.

3. Add the leeks and sauté the leeks, while stirring, for about 5 minutes until turn softened.

4. Take a mixing bowl, whisk the eggs. Add the salt, garlic powder, and basil; combine well.

5. Add the bowl mixture over the leeks; stir-cook for 4-5 minutes.

6. Add the spinach and mushrooms; combine the mixture. Season with black pepper.

7. Transfer the skillet/saucepan to the oven. Bake for 10 minutes, or until the eggs are cooked well.

8. Divide into serving plates and serve warm.

Nutritional Values (Per Serving):

Calories 264, Fat 16g, Carbohydrates 17g, Fiber 3g, Protein 19g

Cinnamon Banana Pancakes

Recipe Time: 15 minutes

Serving Size: 2

Diet Type: Gluten Free, Dairy Free, Soy Free, Nut Free

Ingredients:

- 2 eggs
- 1 egg white
- 1 cup rolled oats
- 1 ripe banana, peeled
- 2 teaspoons ground cinnamon
- 1 teaspoon vanilla extract
- ½ teaspoon salt
- 1 tablespoon coconut oil

Cooking Instructions:

1. In a blender, add the oats and grind to make a coarse flour. Add the egg white, banana, eggs, cinnamon, vanilla, and salt. Blend to make a smooth batter.
2. In a skillet (you can also use a saucepan); heat ½ tablespoon oil over medium stove flame.
3. Add half the batter into the pan to spread evenly. Cook for about 2 minutes until small bubbles form. Flip and cook the other side for about 2 minutes.
4. Repeat the same with remaining batter and serve warm.

Nutritional Values (Per Serving):

Calories 248, Fat 7g, Carbohydrates 31g, Fiber 8g, Protein 12g

Ginger Spiced Oats

Recipe Time: 15-20 minutes

Serving Size: 4

Diet Type: Gluten Free, Dairy Free, Soy Free, Nut Free, Vegan, Vegetarian

Ingredients:

- ¼ teaspoon coriander, ground
- 1 ½ tablespoons cinnamon powder
- ¼ teaspoon cloves, ground
- 1 cup oats, steel cut
- 4 cups water
- ¼ teaspoon allspice, ground
- ¼ teaspoon cardamom, ground
- ¼ teaspoon ginger, grated
- A pinch of nutmeg, ground

Cooking Instructions:

1. In a skillet (you can also use a saucepan); heat the water over medium stove flame.
2. Add the oats and stir the mix.
3. Add the cloves, ginger, allspice, coriander, cinnamon, cardamom and nutmeg, stir, cook for 15 minutes.
4. Add into bowls and serve warm.

Nutritional Values (Per Serving):

Calories 179, Fat 3g, Carbohydrates 13g, Fiber 5g, Protein 6g

Turmeric Cinnamon Hot Milk

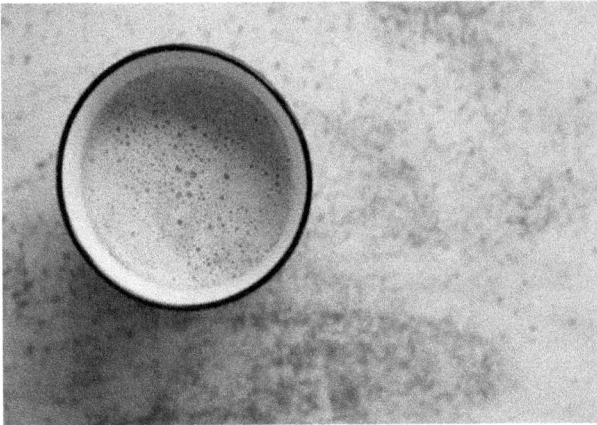

Recipe Time: 5 minutes

Serving Size:2

Diet Type: Gluten Free, Dairy Free, Soy Free, Vegan, Vegetarian

Ingredients:

- ¼ teaspoon ginger, ground
- 1 ½ teaspoon turmeric powder
- 1 ½ cups coconut milk
- 1 ½ cups almond milk
- 1 tablespoon coconut oil
- ¼ teaspoon cinnamon powder

Cooking Instructions:

1. In a skillet (you can also use a saucepan); heat the milks over medium stove flame.

2. Add the ginger, oil, turmeric and cinnamon; stir and cook for 5 minutes.

3. Serve warm.

Nutritional Values (Per Serving):

Calories 168, Fat 3g, Carbohydrates 7g, Fiber 4g, Protein 6g

Cheddar Spinach Frittata

Recipe Time: 35 minutes

Serving Size: 4

Diet Type: Gluten Free, Soy Free

Ingredients:

- ¼ cup coconut milk
- 1 yellow onion, chopped
- 4 ounces white mushrooms, (cut into slices)
- 2 tablespoons olive oil
- 2 cups chopped spinach
- 1 cup cheddar cheese, (shredded or grated)
- 6 eggs
- A pinch of (ground) black pepper and salt

Cooking Instructions:

1. In a skillet (you can also use a saucepan); heat the oil over medium stove flame.
2. Add the onions, stir the mixture and cook while stirring for about 3 minutes until softened.
3. Add the mushrooms, salt and pepper, stir and cook for 2 minutes more.
4. In a bowl (medium size), mix the eggs, cheese, pepper, and salt. Add the mix over the mushrooms.
5. Add the spinach, toss the mixture.
6. Preheat an oven to 360°F.

7. Add the skillet to the oven and bake for 25 minutes. Slice and serve the frittata.

Nutritional Values (Per Serving):

Calories 204, Fat 3g, Carbohydrates 16g, Fiber 6g, Protein 6g

Quinoa Blueberry Bowl

Recipe Time: 5 minutes

Serving Size: 2

Diet Type: Gluten Free, Dairy Free, Soy Free, Vegetarian

Ingredients:

- 2 cups quinoa, cooked
- ¼ cup walnuts, chopped and toasted
- 1 cup cashew or almond milk, warm
- 1 cup blueberries
- 2 teaspoons raw honey
- ½ teaspoon cinnamon powder
- 1 tablespoon chia seeds

Cooking Instructions:

1. In a bowl (medium size), mix the warm milk with the walnuts, honey, blueberries, quinoa, cinnamon and chia seeds.
2. Combine well.
3. Add into serving bowls and serve.

Nutritional Values (Per Serving):

Calories 146, Fat 2g, Carbohydrates 14g, Fiber 5g, Protein 6g

Classic Banana Almond Pancakes

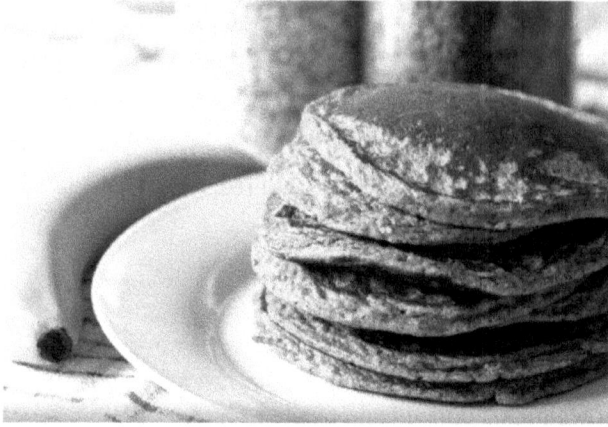

Recipe Time: 10-15 minutes

Serving Size: 4

Diet Type: Gluten Free, Dairy Free, Soy Free

Ingredients:

- 1 teaspoon baking soda
- 3 eggs, beaten
- ½ cup almond flour
- ¼ cup coconut flour
- 2 bananas, peeled and mashed
- 1 teaspoon pure vanilla extract
- 1 tablespoon coconut oil
- Pure maple syrup to taste (optional)

Cooking Instructions:

1. In a bowl (medium size), combine together the flours, and baking soda until well mixed.

2. Make a well in the center and add the bananas, eggs, and vanilla. Combine the mix again.

3. In a skillet (you can also use a saucepan); heat $1/4^{th}$ oil over medium stove flame.

4. Pour ¼ cup of batter and spread evenly.

5. Cook for about 3 minutes, until bubbles form on the surface. Flip and cook for about 2 minutes more.

    Repeat with the remaining batter. Serve with a drizzle of maple syrup.

Nutritional Values (Per Serving):

Calories 127, Fat 7g, Carbohydrates 9g, Fiber 3g, Protein 5g

Apple Oats Granola

Recipe Time: 45 minutes

Serving Size: 6

Diet Type: Gluten Free, Dairy Free, Soy Free, Nut Free, Vegan, Vegetarian

Ingredients:

- 1 cup sunflower seeds
- 1 cup pumpkin seeds
- 2 cups oats
- 1 cup buckwheat
- 1cup apple puree
- 1 ½ cups dates, pitted and chopped
- 6 tablespoons coconut oil
- 5 tablespoons cocoa powder
- 1 teaspoon ginger, (shredded or grated)

Cooking Instructions:

1. Preheat an oven to 360°F.
2. In a mixing bowl, mix the dates, apple puree, oil, buckwheat, oats, seeds, cocoa powder and ginger.
3. Add over a lined baking sheet, press well to make it of even thickness.
4. Bake for 45 minutes or until cooks well.
5. Slice and serve warm.

Nutritional Values (Per Serving):

Calories 168, Fat 3g, Carbohydrates 12g, Fiber 3g, Protein 7g

Coconut Crepes

Recipe Time: 20-25 minutes

Serving Size: 4

Diet Type: Gluten Free, Dairy Free, Soy Free

Ingredients:

- ½ cup almond milk
- ½ cup water
- 2 eggs
- 1 teaspoon vanilla extract
- 2 tablespoons maple syrup or agave nectar
- 1 cup coconut flour
- 3 tablespoons coconut oil

Cooking Instructions:

1. In a bowl (medium size), mix the eggs. Add the vanilla extract, milk, water and sweetener, and whisk well.
2. Add the flour and 1 tablespoon oil; combine to make a smooth batter.
3. In a skillet (you can also use a saucepan); heat ¼ tablespoon oil over medium stove flame.
4. Pour ¼ cup of batter and spread evenly.
5. Cook until turns light brown. Flip and cook until turns light brown. Repeat with the remaining batter.

Nutritional Values (Per Serving):

Calories 132, Fat 3g, Carbohydrates 13g, Fiber 5g, Protein 6g

Strawberry Chia Breakfast

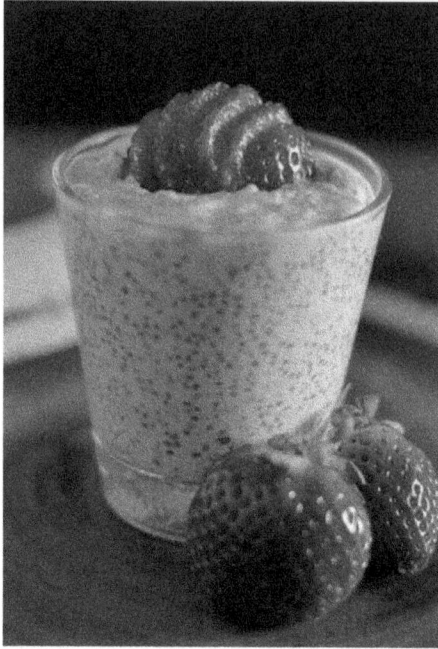

Recipe Time: 30 minutes

Serving Size: 4

Diet Type: Gluten Free, Dairy Free, Soy Free, Vegetarian

Ingredients:

- 1 teaspoon pure vanilla extract
- ¼ cup chia seeds
- ¼ cup shredded coconut, unsweetened
- ¾ cup water
- ¾ cup unsweetened almond milk

- 2 tablespoons raw honey
- ½ cup strawberries, sliced

Cooking Instructions:

1. In a bowl (medium size), whisk the water, milk, and vanilla.
2. Add the chia seeds, and mix well. Cover the bowl, and refrigerate for 30 minutes or overnight.
3. Mix in the coconut and honey.
4. Add the porridge into serving bowls. Serve topped with the strawberries.

Nutritional Values (Per Serving):

Calories 123, Fat 7g, Carbohydrates 14g, Fiber 5g, Protein 2g

Pepper Egg Breakfast

Recipe Time: 5 minutes

Serving Size: 2

Diet Type: Gluten Free, Dairy Free, Soy Free, Nut Free

Ingredients:

- A pinch of garlic powder
- A pinch of (ground) black pepper and salt
- 1 tablespoon olive oil
- ½ cup yellow onions, chopped
- ½ cup red bell pepper, chopped
- 2 eggs

Cooking Instructions:

1. In a skillet (you can also use a saucepan); heat the oil over medium stove flame.
2. Add the onions, stir the mixture and cook while stirring for about 2-3 minutes until softened.
3. Add the bell pepper, garlic powder, salt and pepper, stir and cook for 2-3 minutes more.
4. Add the eggs, stir-cook until the eggs are cooked well.
5. Serve warm.

Nutritional Values (Per Serving):

Calories 216, Fat 6g, Carbohydrates 14g, Fiber 7g, Protein 11g

Hemp Chia Porridge

Recipe Time: 15 minutes

Serving Size: 2

Diet Type: Gluten Free, Dairy Free, Soy Free, Vegan, Vegetarian

Ingredients:

- 2 tablespoons chia seeds
- 1 cup almond milk
- ¼ cup coconut milk
- ¼ cup walnuts, chopped and toasted
- 2 tablespoons hemp seeds, toasted
- ¼ cup coconut, shredded and toasted
- 1 tablespoon coconut oil
- ¼ cup almond butter
- ½ teaspoon turmeric powder
- A pinch of black pepper

Cooking Instructions:

1. In a skillet (you can also use a saucepan); heat the milks over medium stove flame.
2. Add the walnuts, seeds, coconut, turmeric, black pepper; stir-cook for 4-5 minutes.
3. Add the coconut oil and the almond butter, stir the mix and cool down for 5 minutes.
4. Serve and enjoy.

Nutritional Values (Per Serving):

Calories 148, Fat 11g, Carbohydrates 16g, Fiber 6g, Protein 11g

Kale Pistachio Smoothie

Recipe Time: 5 minutes

Serving Size: 2

Diet Type: Gluten Free, Dairy Free, Soy Free, Vegan, Vegetarian

Ingredients:

- 2 frozen bananas, cut into chunks
- ½ cup shelled pistachios
- 1 cup almond milk, unsweetened
- 1 cup shredded kale
- 2 tablespoons pure maple syrup
- 1 teaspoon pure vanilla extract
- 3-4 ice cubes (optional)

Cooking Instructions:

1. Take a high-speed blender (you can also use a food processor) and open top lid.
2. Add the milk and other ingredients. Ice cubes are optional to add (add them if you like your smoothie chilled.)
3. Blend the ingredients over high speed to make a smoothie like texture.
4. Add the blended mixture in glasses and enjoy the fresh smoothie.

Nutritional Values (Per Serving):

Calories 278, Fat 4g, Carbohydrates 41g, Fiber 5g, Protein 6g

Mint Summer Smoothie

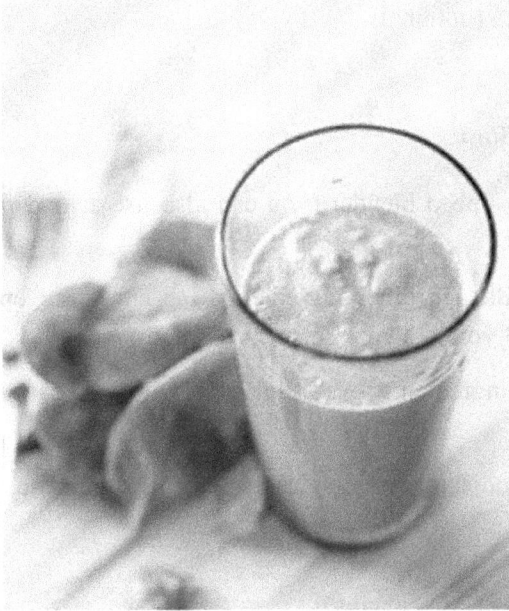

Recipe Time: 5 minutes

Serving Size: 2

Diet Type: Gluten Free, Dairy Free, Soy Free, Nut Free, Vegetarian

Ingredients:

- 1 banana, cut into chunks

- ½ avocado

- 1 cup coconut milk

- 1 cup fresh spinach leaves

- ½ English cucumber, cut into chunks

- 2 tablespoons chopped fresh mint

- 1 tablespoon lemon juice

- 1 tablespoon raw honey

- 3-4 ice cubes (optional)

Cooking Instructions:

1. Take a high-speed blender (you can also use a food processor) and open top lid.

2. Add the milk and other ingredients. Ice cubes are optional to add (add them if you like your smoothie chilled.)

3. Blend the ingredients over high speed to make a smoothie like texture.

4. Add the blended mixture in glasses and enjoy the fresh smoothie.

Nutritional Values (Per Serving):

Calories 384, Fat 21g, Carbohydrates 32g, Fiber 9g, Protein 6g

Fig Yogurt Smoothie

Recipe Time: 5 minutes

Serving Size: 2

Diet Type: Gluten Free, Dairy Free, Soy Free, Vegetarian

Ingredients:

- 1 cup plain whole-milk yogurt
- 1 cup almond milk
- 6-7 whole figs, halved
- 1 banana, cut into chunks
- 1 tablespoon almond butter (optional)
- 1 teaspoon ground flaxseed
- 1 teaspoon raw honey
- Ice cubes (optional)

Cooking Instructions:

1. Take a high-speed blender (you can also use a food processor) and open top lid.
2. Add the milk, yogurt and other ingredients. Ice cubes are optional to add (add them if you like your smoothie chilled.)
3. Blend the ingredients over high speed to make a smoothie like texture.
4. Add the blended mixture in glasses and enjoy the fresh smoothie.

Nutritional Values (Per Serving):

Calories 258, Fat 2g, Carbohydrates 48g, Fiber 9g, Protein 8g

Avocado Cocoa Smoothie

Recipe Time: 5 minutes

Serving Size: 2

Diet Type: Gluten Free, Dairy Free, Soy Free, Vegetarian

Ingredients:

- ½ avocado, pitted and halved
- ½ banana, cut into chunks
- 1 cup unsweetened almond milk
- 1 cup shredded kale
- 1 tablespoon coconut oil
- 1 tablespoon raw honey
- 1 teaspoon pure vanilla extract
- 2 tablespoons cocoa powder
- 4 ice cubes

Cooking Instructions:

1. Take a high-speed blender (you can also use a food processor) and open top lid.
2. Add the milk and other ingredients. Ice cubes are optional to add (add them if you like your smoothie chilled.)
3. Blend the ingredients over high speed to make a smoothie like texture.
4. Add the blended mixture in glasses and enjoy the fresh smoothie.

Nutritional Values (Per Serving):

Calories 286, Fat 19g, Carbohydrates 25g, Fiber 5g, Protein 3g

Pumpkin Cinnamon Smoothie

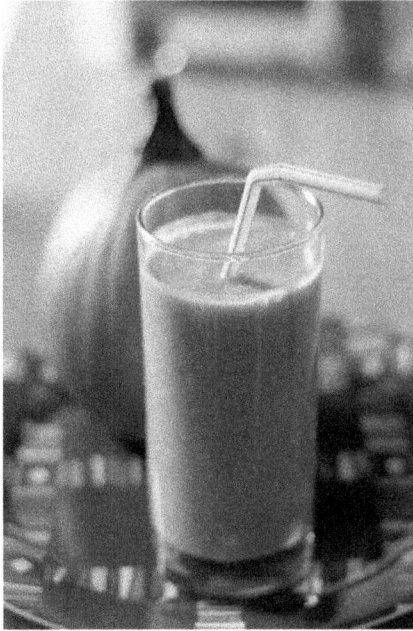

Recipe Time: 5 minutes

Serving Size: 2

Diet Type: Gluten Free, Dairy Free, Soy Free, Vegan, Vegetarian

Ingredients:

- 1 tablespoon maple syrup
- 1 teaspoon (shredded or grated) ginger
- 1 cup unsweetened almond milk
- 1 cup pumpkin purée
- ¼ teaspoon ground cinnamon

- ⅛ teaspoon ground nutmeg

- Pinch ground cloves

- Pinch ground cardamom

- 4 ice cubes

Cooking Instructions:

1. Take a high-speed blender (you can also use a food processor) and open top lid.

2. Add the milk and other ingredients. Ice cubes are optional to add (add them if you like your smoothie chilled.)

3. Blend the ingredients over high speed to make a smoothie like texture.

4. Add the blended mixture in glasses and enjoy the fresh smoothie.

Nutritional Values (Per Serving):

Calories 84, Fat 2g, Carbohydrates 17g, Fiber 4g, Protein 2g

Carrot Pineapple Juice

Recipe Time: 5 minutes

Serving Size: 2

Diet Type: Gluten Free, Dairy Free, Soy Free, Nut Free, Vegan, Vegetarian

Ingredients:

- 8 carrots, peeled and chopped
- 3 cups chopped fresh pineapple
- ¼ cup water
- 1 (1-inch) piece peeled ginger
- Ice cubes, for serving

Cooking Instructions:

1. Take a high-speed blender (you can also use a food processor) and open top lid.
2. Add the milk and other ingredients.
3. Blend the ingredients over high speed to make a smooth mix.
4. Strain the mixture using a cheesecloth in a large bowl. Squeeze through the cheesecloth.
5. Pour the strained mixture in glasses, add the ice cubes (optional) and enjoy the fresh juice.

Nutritional Values (Per Serving):

Calories 124, Fat 1g, Carbohydrates 38g, Fiber 2g, Protein 3g

Cherry Beet Smoothie

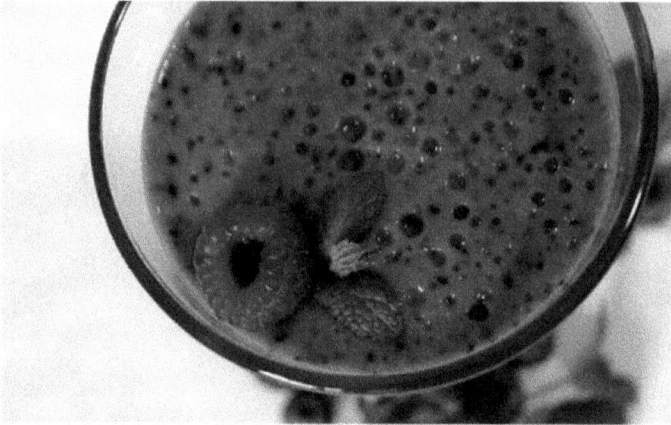

Recipe Time: 5 minutes

Serving Size: 2

Diet Type: Gluten Free, Dairy Free, Soy Free, Vegan, Vegetarian

Ingredients:

- ½ banana, cut into chunks
- ½ cup cherries, pitted
- 10 ounces almond milk
- 2 beets, peeled and cut into small chunks
- 1 tablespoon almond butter
- 3-4 ice cubes (optional)

Cooking Instructions:

1. Take a high-speed blender (you can also use a food processor) and open top lid.

2. Add the milk and other ingredients. Ice cubes are optional to add (add them if you like your smoothie chilled.)

3. Blend the ingredients over high speed to make a smoothie like texture.

4. Add the blended mixture in glasses and enjoy the fresh smoothie.

Nutritional Values (Per Serving):

Calories 156, Fat 5g, Carbohydrates 12g, Fiber 5g, Protein 6g

Pineapple Lush Red Smoothie

Recipe Time: 5 minutes

Serving Size: 2

Diet Type: Gluten Free, Dairy Free, Soy Free, Nut Free, Vegan, Vegetarian

Ingredients:

- 1 banana, cut into chunks
- ½ cup fresh raspberries
- 1 cup coconut water
- ½ cup unsweetened pineapple juice
- ½ cup unsweetened shredded coconut
- 3-4 ice cubes

Cooking Instructions:

1. Take a high-speed blender (you can also use a food processor) and open top lid.
2. Add the coconut water and other ingredients. Ice cubes are optional to add (add them if you like your smoothie chilled.)
3. Blend the ingredients over high speed to make a smoothie like texture.
4. Add the blended mixture in glasses and enjoy the fresh smoothie.

Nutritional Values (Per Serving):

Calories 214, Fat 9g, Carbohydrates 28g, Fiber 7g, Protein 3g

Appetizers
&
Sides

Potato Zucchini Appetizers

Recipe Time: 30 minutes

Serving Size: 4

Diet Type: Gluten Free, Dairy Free, Soy Free, Nut Free, Vegan, Vegetarian

Ingredients:

- 1 yellow bell pepper, diced into small bite size
- 2 zucchini, diced into small bite size
- 1 red bell pepper, diced into small bite size
- 1 red onion, diced into small bite size
- 1 sweet potato, diced into small bite size
- 4 garlic cloves
- ¼ cup extra-virgin olive oil
- 1 teaspoon salt

Cooking Instructions:

1. Preheat an oven to 450°F. Line a baking sheet with a foil.
2. In a mixing bowl, combine the zucchini, red bell pepper, yellow bell pepper, onion, olive oil, sweet potato, garlic, and salt.
3. Arrange evenly on the sheet.
4. Bake for 25 minutes, stirring halfway through. Serve warm.

Nutritional Values (Per Serving):

Calories 176, Fat 12g, Carbohydrates 16g, Fiber 3g, Protein 2g

Spinach Stuffed Mushrooms

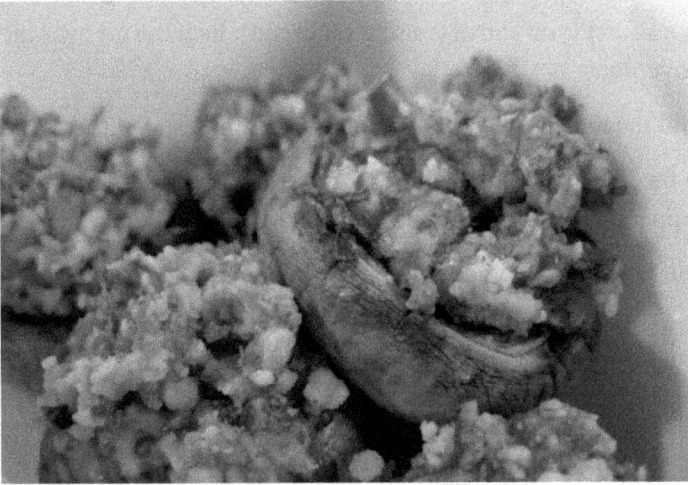

Recipe Time: 35-40 minutes

Serving Size: 12

Diet Type: Gluten Free, Dairy Free, Soy Free, Nut Free, Vegan, Vegetarian

Ingredients:

- 2 pounds button mushrooms, stems reserved
- 3 garlic cloves, minced
- 2 cups spinach, chopped
- 1 tablespoon olive oil
- 2 small red bell peppers, chopped
- 1 small yellow onion, chopped
- (ground) black pepper and salt to the taste
- ¼ cup parsley, chopped

Cooking Instructions:

1. Preheat an oven to 350°F. Line a baking sheet with a foil.

2. In a skillet (you can also use a saucepan); heat the oil over medium stove flame.

3. Add the mushroom, stir and cook for 2 minutes. Set them aside.

4. In the skillet, add the bell peppers, garlic, parsley, spinach, salt, pepper and onion; stir-cook for 5-6 minutes.

5. Stuff each mushroom with the spinach mix.

6. Place them on a lined baking sheet; bake for 20 minutes and serve warm.

Nutritional Values (Per Serving):

Calories 132, Fat 8g, Carbohydrates 9g, Fiber 4g, Protein 9g

Baked Beet Sides

Recipe Time: 30 minutes

Serving Size: 6

Diet Type: Gluten Free, Dairy Free, Soy Free, Nut Free, Vegetarian

Ingredients:

- ½ yellow onion, sliced
- 4 medium golden beets, peeled and diced into small bite size
- 4 medium red beets, peeled and diced into small bite size
- ½ cup apple cider vinegar
- ½ cup extra-virgin olive oil
- 2 tablespoons raw honey
- ¼ teaspoon salt
- Freshly ground black pepper

Cooking Instructions:

1. Preheat an oven to 450°F. Line a baking sheet with a foil.
2. Arrange the beets and onion; drizzle with the vinegar, honey and olive oil.
3. Sprinkle the pepper and salt.
4. Bake for 25 minutes, or until the beets caramelize.
5. Serve warm.

Nutritional Values (Per Serving):

Calories 228, Fat 18g, Carbohydrates 16g, Fiber 3g, Protein 2g

Sesame Bok Choy Side

Recipe Time: 20 minutes

Serving Size: 4

Diet Type: Gluten Free, Dairy Free, Soy Free, Nut Free, Vegan, Vegetarian

Ingredients:

- 1-inch ginger, (shredded or grated)
- 2 tablespoons olive oil
- 3 tablespoons coconut aminos
- A pinch of red pepper flakes
- 4 bok choy heads, cut into quarters
- 2 garlic cloves, minced
- 1 tablespoon sesame seeds, toasted

Cooking Instructions:

1. In a skillet (you can also use a saucepan); heat the oil over medium stove flame.
2. Add the coconut aminos, garlic, pepper flakes and ginger; stir-cook for 4 minutes.
3. Add the bok choy and sesame seeds, toss, cook for 5-6 minutes. Serve warm.

Nutritional Values (Per Serving):

Calories , Fat g, Carbohydrates g, Fiber g, Protein g

Salmon Bites

Recipe Time: 25-30 minutes

Serving Size: 2

Diet Type: Gluten Free, Dairy Free, Soy Free, Nut Free

Ingredients:

- 2 teaspoons garlic powder

- 1 teaspoon onion powder

- 20 ounces canned pineapple pieces

- ½ teaspoon ginger, (shredded or grated)

- 1 tablespoon balsamic vinegar

- 2 salmon fillets, boneless, skinless and cubed

- Black pepper to the taste

Cooking Instructions:

1. Preheat an oven to 375°F. Grease a baking dish with some cooking spray.

2. Place the salmon and pineapple in the dish.

3. Add the ginger, garlic powder, onion powder, black pepper and vinegar, toss the mix.

4. Bake for 20 minutes, divide into bowls and serve.

Nutritional Values (Per Serving):

Calories 198, Fat 2g, Carbohydrates 8g, Fiber 3g, Protein 14g

Garlic Cauliflower

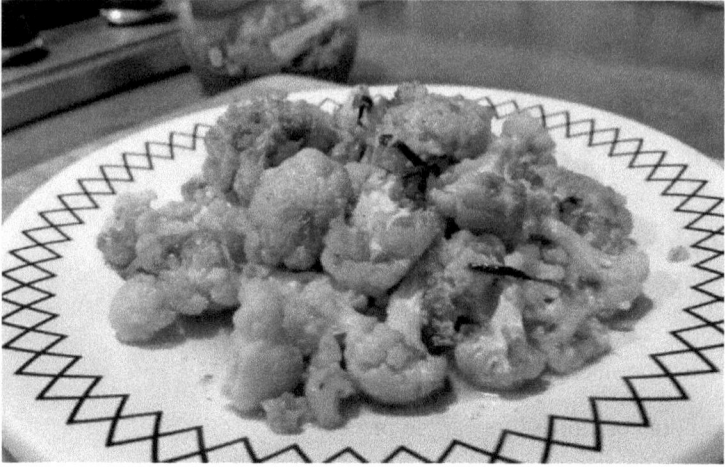

Recipe Time: 15-20 minutes

Serving Size: 4

Diet Type: Gluten Free, Soy Free, Nut Free, Vegetarian

Ingredients:

- ½ teaspoon freshly ground black pepper
- ½ teaspoon garlic powder
- 1½ teaspoons ground cumin
- 1 teaspoon salt
- ½ teaspoon chili powder
- 1 head cauliflower, chopped into bite-size pieces
- 3 tablespoons lime juice
- 3 tablespoons ghee

Cooking Instructions:

1. Preheat an oven to 450°F. Grease a baking dish with some cooking spray.

2. In a bowl, mix the cumin, salt, chili powder, pepper, and garlic powder.

3. Spread the cauliflower in the pan. Drizzle with the lime juice and ghee.

4. Top with the spice mixture and toss to coat.

5. Bake for 15 minutes and serve warm.

Nutritional Values (Per Serving):

Calories 136, Fat 11g, Carbohydrates 9g, Fiber 3g, Protein 4g

Lentil Potato Patties

Recipe Time: 20 minutes

Serving Size: 7-8

Diet Type: Gluten Free, Dairy Free, Soy Free, Vegan, Vegetarian

Ingredients:

- 1 cup canned red lentils, drained and mashed
- 1 sweet potato, (shredded or grated)
- ¼ cup parsley, chopped
- 2 teaspoons ginger, (shredded or grated)
- 1 cup yellow onion, chopped
- 1 cup mushrooms, minced
- 1 tablespoon curry powder
- ¼ cup cilantro, chopped
- 2 tablespoons coconut flour
- 1 tablespoon olive oil

Cooking Instructions:

1. Add the onion, ginger, mushrooms, lentils, potato, curry powder, parsley, cilantro and flour in a bowl.
2. Combine well and prepare patties out of this mix.
3. In a skillet (you can also use a saucepan); heat the oil over medium stove flame.
4. Add the patties and cook for about 5 minutes on each side and serve warm.

Nutritional Values (Per Serving):

Calories 136, Fat 4g, Carbohydrates 7g, Fiber 3g, Protein 8g

Garlic Tomato Sides

Recipe Time: 25 minutes

Serving Size: 6

Diet Type: Gluten Free, Dairy Free, Soy Free, Nut Free, Vegan, Vegetarian

Ingredients:

- 4 garlic cloves, minced
- 1 pound cherry tomatoes, halved
- 1 teaspoon dried basil (optional)
- 2 tablespoons extra-virgin olive oil
- Salt to taste

Cooking Instructions:

1. Preheat an oven to 400°F. Line a baking sheet with a foil.
2. In a bowl, mix the tomatoes, garlic, and basil. Add the olive oil and toss to coat well. Season generously with salt.
3. Add the mix to the sheet.
4. Bake for 15-20 minutes, or until the tomatoes are cooked well.
5. Serve warm.

Nutritional Values (Per Serving):

Calories 47, Fat 0g, Carbohydrates 9g, Fiber 3g, Protein 2g

Awesome Asparagus

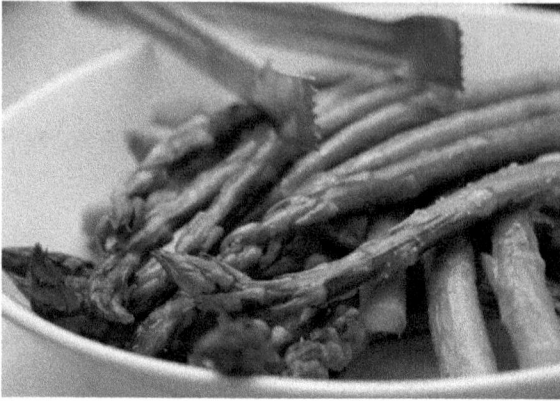

Recipe Time: 25 minutes

Serving Size: 4

Diet Type: Gluten Free, Dairy Free, Soy Free, Nut Free, Vegan, Vegetarian

Ingredients:

- 2 tablespoons shallot, chopped
- 5 tablespoons olive oil
- 4 garlic cloves, minced
- Black pepper to the taste
- 1 ½ teaspoons balsamic vinegar
- 1 ½ pound asparagus, trimmed

Cooking Instructions:

1. Preheat an oven to 450°F. Line a baking sheet with a foil.
2. Spread the asparagus on the sheet.

70

3. Top with the remaining ingredients and coat well.

4. Bake for 15 minutes and serve warm.

Nutritional Values (Per Serving):

Calories 124, Fat 1g, Carbohydrates 4g, Fiber 2g, Protein 3g

Garlic Kale Sides

Recipe Time: 25 minutes

Serving Size: 4

Diet Type: Gluten Free, Dairy Free, Soy Free, Nut Free, Vegan, Vegetarian

Ingredients:

- 8 cups chopped kale
- 1 tablespoon olive oil
- 3 garlic cloves, crushed
- 1 tablespoon balsamic vinegar
- ½ teaspoon ground nutmeg
- Sea salt to taste

Cooking Instructions:

1. In a skillet (you can also use a saucepan); heat the oil over medium stove flame.
2. Add the garlic, stir the mixture and cook while stirring for about 3-4 minutes until fragrant.
3. Add the kale; stir-cook for about 5-7 minutes, or until wilted.
4. Stir in the balsamic vinegar; sprinkle with nutmeg, and sea salt.
5. Serve warm.

Nutritional Values (Per Serving):

Calories 98, Fat 4g, Carbohydrates 14g, Fiber 3g, Protein 4g

Soups & Stews

Chicken Veggie Dinner Soup

Recipe Time: 55-60 minutes

Serving Size: 6-7

Meal Type: Dinner

Diet Type: Gluten Free, Dairy Free, Soy Free, Nut Free

Ingredients:

- 2 teaspoons minced garlic
- 3 cups shredded fennel
- 3 cups shredded green cabbage
- 1 tablespoon olive oil
- 1 sweet onion, chopped
- 2 carrots, chopped
- 8 cups chicken bone broth
- 2 teaspoons chopped fresh thyme
- 2 cups cooked chicken breast, chopped
- Pinch sea salt to taste

Cooking Instructions:

1. In a cooking pot (you can also use a deep saucepan); heat the oil over medium stove flame.

2. Add the onions, garlic, stir the mixture and cook while stirring for about 2-3 minutes until softened.

3. Stir in the fennel, cabbage, and carrots. Sauté for about 4-5 minutes.

4. Stir in the broth and thyme. Bring the soup to a boil.

5. Reduce the heat to low and simmer the mixture for 25-30 minutes, or until the veggies are tender.

6. Add the chicken and salt. Stir and simmer for about 5 minutes. Serve warm.

Nutritional Values (Per Serving):

Calories 246, Fat 9g, Carbohydrates 16g, Fiber 5g, Protein 24g

Mushroom Lentil Soup

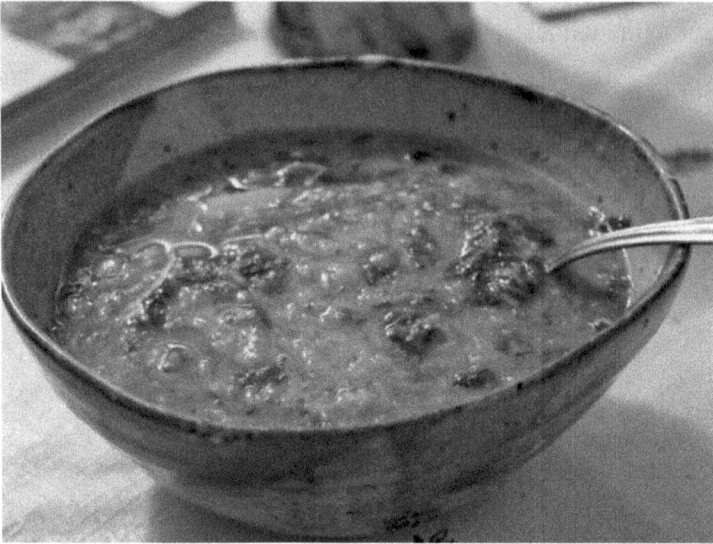

Recipe Time: 30 minutes

Serving Size: 4

Meal Type: Lunch

Diet Type: Gluten Free, Dairy Free, Soy Free, Nut Free, Vegan, Vegetarian

Ingredients:

- 1 medium yellow onion, chopped
- 1 cup white mushrooms, quartered
- 1 1/2 tablespoons coconut oil
- 2 cloves garlic, minced
- 3 cups vegetable broth
- 3 teaspoons miso paste

- 1 cup cooked lentils
- 2 cups kale

Cooking Instructions:

1. In a cooking pot (you can also use a deep saucepan); heat the oil over medium stove flame.
2. Add the garlic, stir the mixture and cook while stirring for about 1 minutes until fragrant.
3. Add the onions and cook for 2-3 minutes until turn soft.
4. Add the mushrooms; stir-cook for another 5 minutes.
5. Add the broth and boil the mixture. Decrease the heat to low flame.
6. Mix in the miso paste and lentils; cook for 5 minute.
7. Stirs in the kale. Let it cook for another 3 minutes.
8. Serve warm.

Nutritional Values (Per Serving):

Calories 294, Fat 4g, Carbohydrates 8g, Fiber 2g, Protein 15g

Pork Chili Stew

Recipe Time: 1 hour 50 minutes

Serving Size: 4-6

Meal Type: Dinner

Diet Type: Gluten Free, Dairy Free, Soy Free, Nut Free

Ingredients:

- 3 tablespoons olive oil
- 3 pounds pork shoulder, cubed
- 2 yellow onions, chopped
- 2 tablespoons garlic, minced
- 2 cups almond flour
- A pinch of (ground) black pepper and salt
- 1 teaspoon chili pepper flakes, dried
- 3 cups chicken stock
- 4 tablespoons sage, chopped
- ¼ cup tomato paste
- ½ teaspoon all-spice

Cooking Instructions:

1. In a bowl (medium size), mix the flour, salt and pepper.

2. Coat the pork in this mix.

3. In a cooking pot (you can also use a deep saucepan); heat the oil over medium stove flame.

4. Add the meat and cook, while stirring, until becomes evenly brown.

5. Transfer it to a bowl.

6. In the pan, add the garlic, onion, sage and pepper flakes and stir-cook for 8 minutes.

7. Add the pork to the pan; mix in the stock, allspice and tomato paste.

8. Stir and cook everything for 80-90 minutes.

9. Divide into serving bowls and serve warm.

Nutritional Values (Per Serving):

Calories 271, Fat 4g, Carbohydrates 11g, Fiber 6g, Protein 18g

Chicken Jalapeno Soup

Recipe Time: 25-30 minutes

Serving Size: 6

Meal Type: Lunch

Diet Type: Gluten Free, Dairy Free, Soy Free, Nut Free

Ingredients:

- 1 tablespoon avocado oil
- 1 jalapeño pepper, seeded and minced
- 6 cups chicken broth
- 1 pound shredded cooked chicken
- 3 garlic cloves, minced
- 1 medium white onion, diced
- 1 (14-ounce) can diced tomatoes with their juice
- 1 (4-ounce) can diced green chiles
- 3 tablespoons lime juice
- ¼ teaspoon cayenne pepper
- Freshly ground black pepper
- 1 teaspoon chili powder
- 1 teaspoon ground cumin
- ½ teaspoon salt
- 1 avocado, pitted and sliced

Cooking Instructions:

1. In a cooking pot (you can also use a deep saucepan); heat the oil over medium stove flame.

2. Add the garlic, onion, and jalapeño pepper; sauté for 4-5 minutes.

3. Add the broth, chicken, tomatoes, chiles, lime juice, chili powder, cumin, salt, cayenne pepper, and black pepper.

4. Stir the mix and bring to a simmer; cook for 10 minutes.

5. Add in serving bowls and too with the slices of avocado and cilantro.

Nutritional Values (Per Serving):

Calories 274, Fat 7g, Carbohydrates 12g, Fiber 4g, Protein 30g

Broccoli Potato Soup

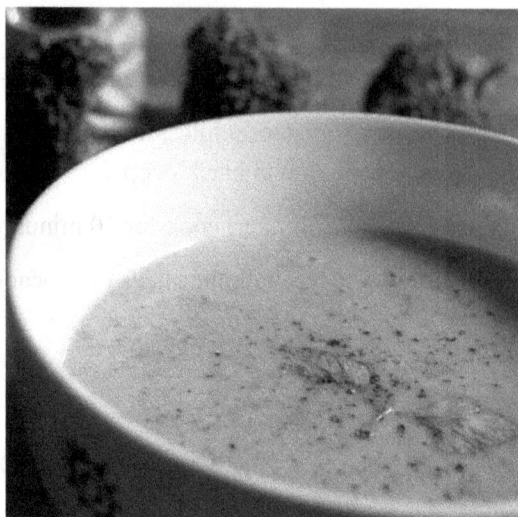

Recipe Time: 40-45 minutes

Serving Size: 6

Meal Type: Lunch

Diet Type: Gluten Free, Dairy Free, Soy Free, Nut Free

Ingredients:

- 1 cup sliced onion
- 2 teaspoons minced garlic
- 1 tablespoon olive oil
- 1 sweet onion, chopped
- 1 sweet potato, peeled and roughly chopped
- 1 teaspoon ground nutmeg

- 8 cups chicken bone broth
- 3 heads broccoli, cut into florets
- ½ cup coconut cream
- Sea salt to taste

Cooking Instructions:

1. In a cooking pot (you can also use a deep saucepan); heat the oil over medium stove flame.
2. Add the onions, garlic, stir the mixture and cook while stirring for about 2-3 minutes until softened.
3. Stir in the broth, broccoli, sweet potato, and nutmeg.
4. Bring it to a boil. Reduce flame to low and simmer for 25-30 minutes, or until the vegetables are tender.
5. Purée the soup in a blender until smooth.
6. Whisk in the cream and season with sea salt. Serve warm.

Nutritional Values (Per Serving):

Calories 184, Fat 9g, Carbohydrates 18g, Fiber 6g, Protein 14g

Tuna Potato Stew

Recipe Time: 40 minutes

Serving Size: 4

Meal Type: Dinner

Diet Type: Gluten Free, Dairy Free, Soy Free, Nut Free

Ingredients:

- 1 teaspoon dried chili
- ¼ pint chicken stock
- 1 yellow onion, chopped
- 1 tablespoon olive oil
- 1 garlic clove, minced
- 14 ounces canned tomatoes, chopped
- 3 sweet potatoes, cubed
- 1 teaspoon sweet paprika
- 2 tuna fillets, flaked
- 1 red pepper, chopped
- 1 tablespoon coriander, chopped

Cooking Instructions:

1. In a cooking pot (you can also use a deep saucepan); heat the oil over medium stove flame.

2. Add the onions, stir the mixture and cook while stirring for about 3-4 minutes until softened.

3. Add the chili and garlic, stir-cook for 1 minute.

4. Add the stock, tomatoes, potatoes, paprika and red pepper, stir the mix.

5. Simmer and cook for 20 minutes over medium flame.

6. Add the tuna, cook for 8-10 minutes.

7. Add into serving bowls, sprinkle coriander on top and serve warm.

Nutritional Values (Per Serving):

Calories 224, Fat 4g, Carbohydrates 16g, Fiber 7g, Protein 7g

Fish Shrimp Soup

Recipe Time: 40 minutes

Serving Size: 6

Meal Type: Dinner

Diet Type: Gluten Free, Dairy Free, Soy Free, Nut Free

Ingredients:

- 2 stalks celery, chopped
- 1 tablespoon olive oil
- 1 sweet onion, chopped
- 2 teaspoons minced garlic
- 2 carrots, diced
- ½ teaspoon ground cumin
- ½ teaspoon ground coriander
- 1 pound haddock, cut into small bite size
- 6 cups chicken bone broth
- 2 cups cubed sweet potato
- ½ pound peeled and deveined shrimp, chopped
- 1 cup chopped spinach
- 2 tablespoons chopped fresh cilantro

Cooking Instructions:

1. In a cooking pot (you can also use a deep saucepan); heat the oil over medium stove flame.

2. Add the onions, garlic, celery, stir the mixture and cook while stirring for about 2-3 minutes until softened.

3. Stir in the broth, sweet potato, carrots, cumin, and coriander.

4. Boil the mix. Reduce flame to low and simmer for about 10 minutes, or until the vegetables are tender.

5. Stir in the haddock and shrimp. Simmer the mix for 8-10 minutes more. Stir in the spinach and simmer for 2 minutes.

6. Add in serving bowls and top with the cilantro.

Nutritional Values (Per Serving):

Calories 244, Fat 8g, Carbohydrates 18g, Fiber 3g, Protein 26g

Yogurt Tomato Soup

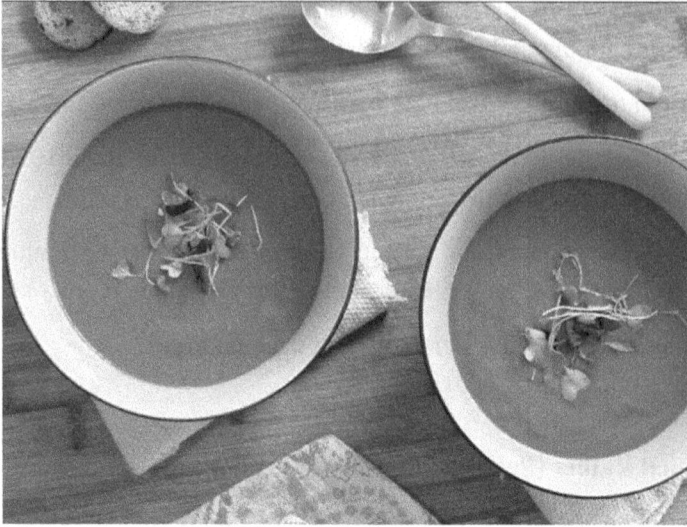

Recipe Time: 25-30 minutes

Serving Size: 6

Meal Type: Lunch

Diet Type: Gluten Free, Soy Free, Nut Free, Vegetarian

Ingredients:

- 1 teaspoon dried basil
- 1 teaspoon dried oregano
- ⅛ teaspoon freshly ground black pepper
- ⅛ teaspoon dried thyme
- ½ teaspoon salt
- ¼ teaspoon chili powder

- 1 tablespoon ghee

- 1 small onion, chopped

- 3 garlic cloves, chopped

- 2 (14-ounce) cans diced tomatoes with their juice

- 2 cups vegetable broth

- ¼ cup tomato paste

- ½ cup plain whole-milk yogurt

Cooking Instructions:

1. In a cooking pot (you can also use a deep saucepan); heat the oil over medium stove flame.

2. Add the onions, garlic, stir the mixture and cook while stirring for about 4-5 minutes until softened.

3. Stir in the basil, oregano, salt, chili powder, pepper, and thyme.

4. Add the tomatoes, broth, and tomato paste; combine well.

5. Bring to a simmer, turn flame to low, and cook for 8-10 minutes.

6. Puree the mix in a blender and add the yogurt. Blend for 1 minute more.

7. Serve warm.

Nutritional Values (Per Serving):

Calories 152, Fat 6g, Carbohydrates 26g, Fiber 12g, Protein 8g

Artichoke Chicken Stew

Recipe Time: 65 minutes

Serving Size: 7-8

Meal Type: Dinner

Diet Type: Gluten Free, Dairy Free, Soy Free, Nut Free

Ingredients:

- 5 garlic cloves, minced
- 2 tablespoons olive oil
- 2 yellow onions, chopped
- 2 pounds chicken thighs, skinless, boneless and chopped
- 1 tablespoon maple syrup
- 2 cups vegetable stock
- 16 ounces canned artichoke hearts, drained and chopped
- A pinch of sea (ground) black pepper and salt
- 2 tablespoons cilantro, chopped

Cooking Instructions:

1. In a cooking pot (you can also use a deep saucepan); heat 1 tablespoon oil over medium stove flame.
2. Add the chicken, and cook, while stirring, until becomes evenly brown.
3. Transfer to a bowl (medium size).

4. In the pan heat the remaining oil, add the garlic and onion, stir and cook for 1 minute.

5. Add the stock, maple syrup, artichokes, salt and pepper, stir the mix.

6. Simmer and cook for 3-4 minutes.

7. Add the chicken to the pot, stir the mix.

8. Cover the pot, reduce flame to low, cook for 45 minutes.

9. Mix in the cilantro and serve warm.

Nutritional Values (Per Serving):

Calories 207, Fat 4g, Carbohydrates 11g, Fiber 4g, Protein 21g

Shrimp Scallops Stew

Recipe Time: 30 minutes

Serving Size: 4

Meal Type: Dinner

Diet Type: Gluten Free, Dairy Free, Soy Free, Nut Free

Ingredients:

- 1 teaspoon jalapeno, chopped
- 2 teaspoons garlic, chopped
- 2 leeks, chopped
- 2 tablespoons olive oil
- 1 carrot, chopped
- 1 teaspoon cumin, ground
- A pinch of (ground) black pepper and salt
- ¼ teaspoon cinnamon powder
- 1 ½ cups tomatoes, chopped
- 1 cup veggie stock
- 1 pound shrimp, peeled and deveined
- 1 pound sea scallops
- 2 tablespoons cilantro, chopped

Cooking Instructions:

1. In a cooking pot (you can also use a deep saucepan); heat the oil over medium stove flame.

2. Add the leek, garlic, stir the mixture and cook while stirring for about 6-7 minutes until softened.

3. Add the jalapeno, salt, pepper, cayenne, carrots, cinnamon and cumin, stir the mix.

4. Cook for 5 minutes. Add the tomatoes, stock, shrimp and scallops, stir the mix.

5. Cook for 5-6 minutes. Add in serving bowls, top with the cilantro and serve warm.

Nutritional Values (Per Serving):

Calories 245, Fat 4g, Carbohydrates 11g, Fiber 5g, Protein 17g

Sprouts Pork Soup

Recipe Time: 25 minutes

Serving Size: 6

Meal Type: Dinner

Diet Type: Gluten Free, Dairy Free, Soy Free, Nut Free

Ingredients:

- 2 tablespoons olive oil
- 5 garlic cloves, minced
- 2 stalks celery, chopped
- ½ pound pork, cubed
- ½ pounds pork, ground
- 3 cups vegetable stock
- 2 scallions, chopped
- Black pepper to the taste
- 1 cup bean sprouts
- 2 tablespoons parsley, chopped
- ½ teaspoon cinnamon powder
- 4 tablespoons coconut aminos
- ½ tablespoon red pepper flakes

Cooking Instructions:

1. In a cooking pot (you can also use a deep saucepan); heat the oil over medium stove flame.

2. Add the pork strips and cook, while stirring, until becomes evenly brown.

3. Transfer to a plate.

4. In the pan, add the garlic, stir and cook for 1-2 minutes.

5. Add the ground pork, pork strips, scallions, celery, stock, black pepper, cinnamon and aminos.

6. Combine well and bring to a boil and cook for 12-15 minutes.

7. Mix in the sprouts, parsley, and pepper flakes, toss well and serve warm.

Nutritional Values (Per Serving):

Calories 296, Fat 4g, Carbohydrates 9g, Fiber 3g, Protein 15g

Chicken White Bean Soup

Recipe Time: 20 minutes

Serving Size: 4

Diet Type: Gluten Free, Dairy Free, Soy Free, Nut Free

Ingredients:

- 2 (4-ounce) cans diced mild green chilies
- 4 cups cooked white beans, drained and rinsed well
- 4 cups chicken broth or vegetable broth
- 1 tablespoon ghee
- 2 small onions, chopped
- 6 garlic cloves, minced
- 1 teaspoon chili powder
- ¼ teaspoon cayenne pepper
- 4 teaspoons ground cumin
- 2 teaspoons dried oregano
- 4 cups shredded cooked chicken
- 2 scallions, (cut into slices)

Cooking Instructions:

1. In a cooking pot (you can also use a deep saucepan); heat the oil over medium stove flame.

2. Add the onions, garlic, stir the mixture and cook while stirring for about 4-5 minutes until softened.

3. Add the chilies, stir-cook for 2 minutes.

4. Stir in the beans, broth, cumin, oregano, chili powder, and cayenne pepper.

5. Simmer the mix and add the chicken. Reduce flame to medium-low, and cook for 8-10 minutes.

6. Top with the scallions and serve warm.

Nutritional Values (Per Serving):

Calories 296, Fat 4g, Carbohydrates 41g, Fiber 12g, Protein 22g

Coconut Avocado Soup

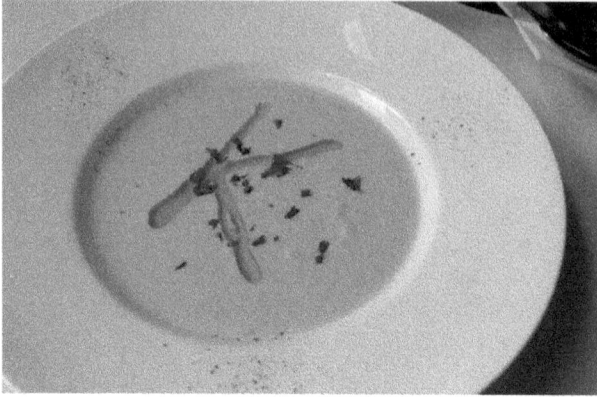

Recipe Time: 15 minutes

Serving Size: 6

Meal Type: Lunch

Diet Type: Gluten Free, Dairy Free, Soy Free, Nut Free, Vegan, Vegetarian

Ingredients:

- 1 tablespoon lemon juice
- 1 garlic clove, crushed
- 1 teaspoon grated ginger
- 3 ripe avocados, peeled and pitted
- ¼ red onion, chopped
- 1 cup chicken bone broth
- ½ teaspoon chopped dill
- 2 cups canned full-fat coconut milk
- Sea salt and ground black pepper to taste

Cooking Instructions:

1. Slice the avocado and set aside.

2. In a blender or food processor, add the avocado, onion, chicken broth, lemon juice, garlic, ginger, and dill. Purée the mixture until very smooth.

3. Transfer in a container. Whisk in the milk. Season with salt and pepper.

4. Chill in your fridge for at least 1 hour.

5. Garnish with the dill sprigs and serve chilled.

Nutritional Values (Per Serving):

Calories 326, Fat 31g, Carbohydrates 14g, Fiber 8g, Protein 4g

Eggplant Pork Stew

Recipe Time: 20 minutes

Serving Size: 4

Meal Type: Dinner

Diet Type: Gluten Free, Dairy Free, Soy Free, Nut Free

Ingredients:

- 4 garlic cloves, minced
- 1 pound pork, ground
- 1 eggplant, cubed
- 2 green onions, chopped
- 2 tablespoons avocado oil
- 14 ounces canned tomatoes, chopped
- (ground) black pepper and salt to the taste
- 1/3 cup basil, chopped
- 2 tablespoons tomato paste
- ¾ cup coconut cream

Cooking Instructions:

1. In a cooking pot (you can also use a deep saucepan); heat the oil over medium stove flame.
2. Add the onions, garlic, stir the mixture and cook while stirring for about 2-3 minutes until softened.
3. Add the beef, stir-cook for 4-5 minutes.
4. Add the eggplant, tomatoes, salt, pepper and basil, stir the mix and cook for 4-5 minutes.
5. Add the tomato paste and cream, stir, cook for 1 minute. Serve warm.

Nutritional Values (Per Serving):

Calories 253, Fat 11g, Carbohydrates 8g, Fiber 1g, Protein 19g

Spinach Mushroom Soup

Recipe Time: 45 minutes

Serving Size: 4

Meal Type: Lunch

Diet Type: Gluten Free, Dairy Free, Soy Free, Nut Free

Ingredients:

- 1 cup sliced mushrooms

- ½ teaspoon fish sauce

- 3 tablespoons miso paste

- 3 cups filtered water

- 3 cups vegetable broth

- 1 cup baby spinach, thoroughly washed

- 4 scallions, (cut into slices)

Cooking Instructions:

1. In a cooking pot (you can also use a deep saucepan); heat the water and broth over medium stove flame.

2. Add the mushrooms, and fish sauce, and boil the mixture. Remove from the heat.

3. In a bowl, mix the miso paste with ½ cup of broth mix. Combine well to dissolve the paste.

4. Add the mix back into the soup. Stir in the spinach and scallions. Serve warm.

Nutritional Values (Per Serving):

Calories 54, Fat 0g, Carbohydrates 9g, Fiber 1g, Protein 2g

Poultry & Chicken

Turkey Green Salad

Recipe Time: 20 minutes

Serving Size: 4

Meal Type: Lunch

Diet Type: Gluten Free, Dairy Free, Soy Free

Ingredients:

Dressing:

- 2 tablespoons balsamic vinegar
- 2 teaspoons Dijon mustard
- ¼ cup olive oil
- 1 teaspoon chopped fresh thyme
- Sea salt to taste

Salad:

- ½ red onion, (cut into slices)
- 4 cups mixed greens
- 1 cup arugula
- 16 ounces cooked turkey breast, chopped
- 3 apricots, pitted and make small pieces
- ½ cup chopped pecans

Cooking Instructions:

1. In a small bowl, whisk the dressing ingredients and set aside.

2. In a salad bowl, add the mixed greens, arugula, and red onion.

3. Top with 3/4 of the dressing.

4. Top with the turkey, apricots, and pecans. Drizzle with the remaining dressing and serve.

Nutritional Values (Per Serving):

Calories 296, Fat 19g, Carbohydrates 12g, Fiber 2g, Protein 21g

Chicken Swiss Salad

Recipe Time: 20 minutes

Serving Size: 6

Meal Type: Lunch

Diet Type: Gluten Free, Dairy Free, Soy Free

Ingredients:

- 4 mini bell peppers, (cut into slices)
- 1 pear, (cut into slices)
- ¼ cup toasted pine nuts
- 2 cups shredded cooked chicken
- 6 cups chopped Swiss chard
- 1 shallot, minced
- ½ cup extra-virgin olive oil
- 2 tablespoons lemon juice
- 2 tablespoons apple cider vinegar
- 1 tablespoon Dijon mustard
- ¼ teaspoon salt

Cooking Instructions:

1. Preheat an oven to 350°F.

2. Wrap the shredded chicken in a piece of aluminum foil; bake for 10 minutes.

3. In a mixing bowl, combine the chard, bell peppers, pear, and nuts.

4. In another bowl, whisk together the shallot, olive oil, lemon juice, vinegar, mustard, and salt.

5. Add the dressing with the nut mix and combine well.

6. Add the baked chicken to the salad. Toss and serve immediately.

Nutritional Values (Per Serving):

Calories 325, Fat 21g, Carbohydrates 9g, Fiber 2g, Protein 14g

Classic Italian Spiced Chicken

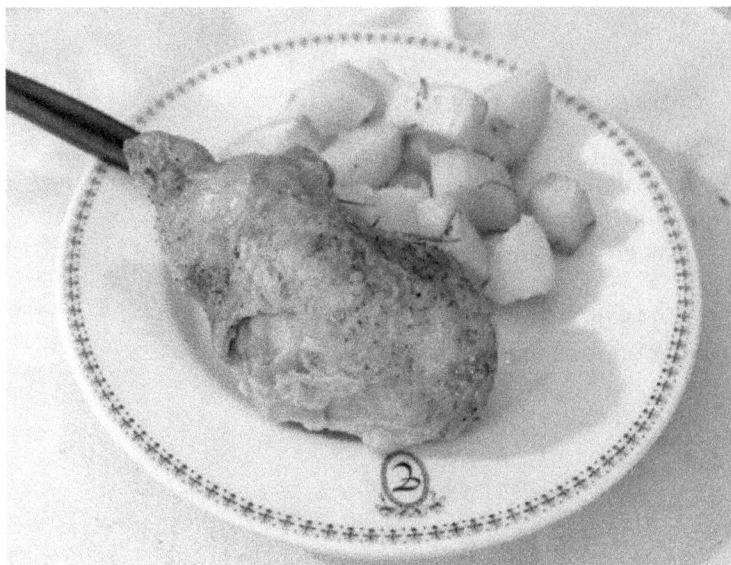

Recipe Time: 70 minutes

Serving Size: 6

Meal Type: Lunch

Diet Type: Gluten Free, Dairy Free, Soy Free, Nut Free

Ingredients:

- 2 tablespoons olive oil

- 1 tablespoon lemon juice

- 1 cup parsley, chopped

- 6 chicken thighs, boneless and skinless

- 2 cups sweet potatoes, cut into wedges

- 2 tablespoons Italian seasoning

Cooking Instructions:

1. Preheat an oven to 450°F. Line a baking sheet with a foil.

2. Add the chicken on a lined sheet; add the potatoes, oil, lemon juice, parsley and seasoning, toss well.

3. Bake the mix for 55-60 minutes until cooked well.

4. Divide between plates and serve.

Nutritional Values (Per Serving):

Calories 236, Fat 7g, Carbohydrates 12g, Fiber 7g, Protein 12g

Chicken Spinach Salad

Recipe Time: 55 minutes

Serving Size: 4

Meal Type: Lunch

Diet Type: Gluten Free, Dairy Free, Soy Free, Nut Free

Ingredients:

- 1 yellow onion, chopped
- 12 ounces mushrooms, chopped
- 2 garlic cloves, minced
- 2 sweet potatoes, baked
- A drizzle of olive oil
- 2 cups baby spinach
- A pinch of salt and cayenne pepper
- ½ teaspoon thyme, dried
- 3 cups chicken, cooked and shredded
- A splash of balsamic vinegar

Cooking Instructions:

1. Cut the potatoes in halves lengthwise; chop into small pieces and add in a bowl (medium size).

2. In a skillet (you can also use a saucepan); heat the oil over medium stove flame.

3. Add the onion, potato pieces, garlic, mushrooms, thyme, chicken, salt and cayenne pepper, toss well.

4.   Cook for 8-10 minutes, take off heat.

5.   Also add the spinach and vinegar, toss and serve.

Nutritional Values (Per Serving):

Calories 263, Fat 2g, Carbohydrates 17g, Fiber 8g, Protein 11g

Brown Rice Chicken Meal

Recipe Time: 20 minutes

Serving Size: 4

Meal Type: Lunch

Diet Type: Gluten Free, Dairy Free, Soy Free, Nut Free

Ingredients:

- 1 ½ cups brown rice, cooked
- 1 ½ tablespoons maple syrup
- 4 ounces chicken breast boneless, skinless and cut into small pieces
- 1 egg
- 2 egg whites
- 1 cup chicken stock
- 2 tablespoon coconut aminos
- 2 scallions, chopped

Cooking Instructions:

1. In a cooking pot (you can also use a deep saucepan); heat the stock over medium stove flame.

2. Add coconut aminos and sugar, stir the mix and boil it.

3. Add the chicken and toss.

4. In a bowl (medium size), whisk the egg with egg whites.

5. Add it over the chicken mix, add the scallions on top and cook for 3 minutes without stirring.

6. Divide into serving bowls and serve.

Nutritional Values (Per Serving):

Calories 246, Fat 11g, Carbohydrates 13g, Fiber 6g, Protein 9g

Turkey Pepper Patties

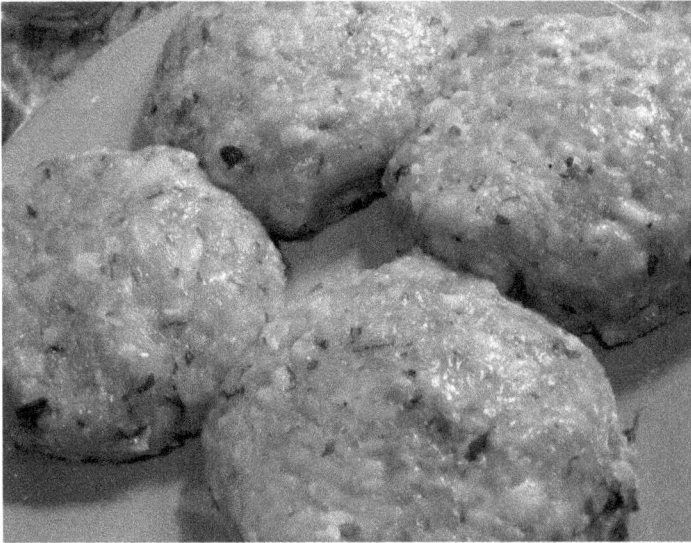

Recipe Time: 20 minutes

Serving Size: 4

Meal Type: Lunch

Diet Type: Gluten Free, Dairy Free, Soy Free, Nut Free

Ingredients:

- 1 pound turkey meat, ground

- 1 small jalapeno pepper, minced

- 2 teaspoons lime juice

- 1 shallot, minced

- 1 tablespoon olive oil

- Zest of 1 lime

- (ground) black pepper and salt to the taste

- 1 teaspoon turmeric powder

Cooking Instructions:

1. In a bowl (medium size), mix the turkey, shallot, jalapeno, lime juice, lime zest, salt, pepper and turmeric.

2. Prepare burger patties from this mix.

3. In a skillet (you can also use a saucepan); heat the oil over medium stove flame.

4. Add the patties and cook them for about 5 minutes on each side.

5. Serve with yogurt dip or green vegetables (optional).

Nutritional Values (Per Serving):

Calories 196, Fat 13g, Carbohydrates 12g, Fiber 5g, Protein 7g

Brussels Chicken Meal

Recipe Time: 20 minutes

Serving Size: 4

Meal Type: Dinner

Diet Type: Gluten Free, Dairy Free, Soy Free

Ingredients:

- 12 ounces Brussels sprouts, shredded
- 1 apple, cored and sliced
- ½ red onion, (cut into slices)
- 1 ½ pounds chicken thighs, skinless and boneless
- 1 tablespoon olive oil
- 2 teaspoons thyme, chopped
- A pinch of (ground) black pepper and salt
- 1 garlic clove, minced
- 2 tablespoons balsamic vinegar
- ¼ cup walnuts, chopped

Cooking Instructions:

1. In a skillet (you can also use a saucepan); heat the oil over medium stove flame.

2. Add the chicken, pepper, salt and thyme; cook, while stirring, until becomes evenly brown.

3. Transfer to a bowl (medium size).

4. In the pan, add the onion, apple, sprouts and garlic, stir-cook for 4-5 minutes.

5. Add the vinegar, cooked chicken, and walnuts, toss, cook for 1-2 minutes.

6. Serve warm.

Nutritional Values (Per Serving):

Calories 223, Fat 4g, Carbohydrates 13g, Fiber 7g, Protein 9g

Broccoli Chicken Light Casserole

Recipe Time: 55 minutes

Serving Size: 4

Meal Type: Lunch

Diet Type: Gluten Free, Dairy Free, Soy Free, Nut Free

Ingredients:

- 8 ounces mushrooms, (cut into slices)
- 3 cups chicken, cooked and shredded
- 4 cups broccoli florets
- 1 yellow onion, chopped
- 2 tablespoons olive oil
- (ground) black pepper and salt to the taste
- 1 cup chicken stock
- ½ teaspoon nutmeg, ground
- 2 eggs

Cooking Instructions:

1. Preheat an oven to 350°F. Grease a baking dish with some cooking spray.
2. In a skillet (you can also use a saucepan); heat the oil over medium stove flame.
3. Add the onions, salt, pepper, mushrooms, stir the mixture and cook while stirring for about 8-10 minutes until softened.
4. Add the mix into a baking dish; mix in the chicken and broccoli

5. In a bowl (medium size), combine the stock, eggs, nutmeg, salt and pepper.

6. Add it over the chicken mix, bake for 40 minutes.

7. Divide between serving plates and serve warm.

Nutritional Values (Per Serving):

Calories 339, Fat 12g, Carbohydrates 13g, Fiber 3g, Protein 16g

Couscous Carrot Chicken

Recipe Time: 30 minutes

Serving Size: 4

Meal Type: Dinner

Diet Type: Dairy Free, Soy Free, Nut Free

Ingredients:

- 1/3 cup roasted pepitas
- 1/3 cup parsley, chopped
- ¼ cup mint, chopped
- 6 ounces couscous, cooked
- 2 teaspoon coconut oil, melted
- 12 ounces baby carrots
- 4 chicken thighs, boneless
- A pinch of (ground) black pepper and salt
- 1 tablespoon lemon juice
- 2 teaspoons lemon zest
- 1 tablespoon olive oil
- 1 garlic clove, minced

Cooking Instructions:

1. Preheat an oven to 450°F. Grease a baking dish with some cooking spray.

2. In a skillet (you can also use a saucepan); heat the oil over medium stove flame.

3. Add the chicken, salt, pepper and cook, while stirring, until becomes evenly brown for 8-10 minutes.

4. Transfer to the baking dish.

5. In the pan, add the carrots and cook for 2-3 minutes.

6. Add the carrots with the chicken; bake for 10 minutes.

7. In a bowl (medium size), mix the couscous, olive oil, salt, pepper, pepitas, parsley, mint, garlic, lemon juice and lemon zest; combine well.

8. Divide the chicken mix between serving plates, add the couscousmix and serve warm.

Nutritional Values (Per Serving):

Calories 264, Fat 4g, Carbohydrates 16g, Fiber 6g, Protein 10g

Turkey Lunch Wraps/Cups

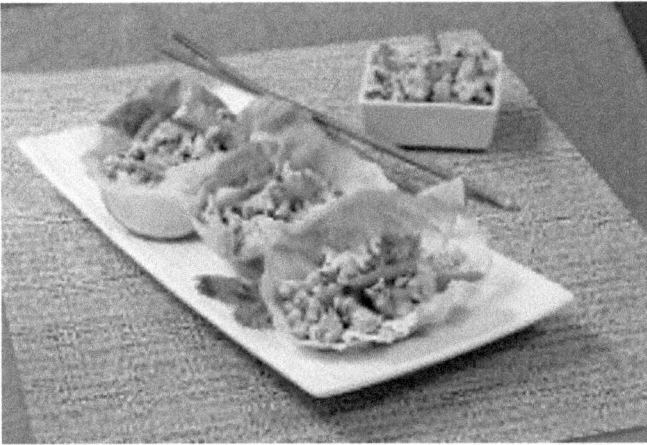

Recipe Time: 25 minutes

Serving Size: 4

Meal Type: Lunch

Diet Type: Gluten Free, Dairy Free, Soy Free, Nut Free

Ingredients:

- 1 pound ground turkey

- 2 tablespoons lime juice

- 2 tablespoons fish sauce

- 2 tablespoons minced cilantro

- 1 tablespoon minced mint (optional)

- 1 tablespoon maple syrup

- 1 small red onion, diced

- 2 garlic cloves, minced

- 4 scallions, (cut into slices)

- ¼ teaspoon red pepper flakes

- 8 small romaine lettuce leaves

Cooking Instructions:

1. In a skillet (you can also use a saucepan); heat the oil over medium stove flame.

2. Add the turkey and cook, while stirring, until becomes evenly brown.

3. Add the onion and garlic, and stir-cook for 8-10 minutes.

4. Remove from the heat.

5. Mix the scallions, lime juice, fish sauce, cilantro, mint, maple syrup, and red pepper flakes; combine well.

6. Add the mix in lettuce leaf. Serve warm.

Nutritional Values (Per Serving):

Calories 153, Fat 2g, Carbohydrates 8g, Fiber 1g, Protein 24g

Spinach Baked Chicken

Recipe Time: 30 minutes

Serving Size: 4

Meal Type: Dinner

Diet Type: Gluten Free, Dairy Free, Soy Free, Nut Free

Ingredients:

- 4 (4-ounce) boneless, skinless chicken breasts
- 1 cup cremini mushrooms, sliced
- ½ red onion, thinly sliced
- ½ cup chopped basil
- 2 tablespoons avocado oil
- 1 pint cherry tomatoes, halved
- 4 garlic cloves, minced
- 2 teaspoons balsamic vinegar
- 1 cup chopped spinach

Cooking Instructions:

1. Preheat an oven to 400°F. Grease a baking dish with some cooking spray.

2. Place the chicken. Brush with the oil.

3. In a bowl (medium size), mix the tomatoes, spinach, mushrooms, red onion, basil, garlic, and vinegar.

4. Top each chicken breast with 1/4th vegetable mixture. Bake for about 18-20 minutes, or until the chicken is cooked well.

5. Serve with the remaining vegetable mix.

Nutritional Values (Per Serving):

Calories 234, Fat 9g, Carbohydrates 8g, Fiber 2g, Protein 27g

Sweet Potato Whole Chicken

Recipe Time: 80-85 minutes

Serving Size: 6

Meal Type: Dinner

Diet Type: Gluten Free, Dairy Free, Soy Free, Nut Free

Ingredients:

- ½ pound sweet potatoes, cubed
- 2 tablespoons olive oil
- 1 whole chicken
- Juice of ½ lemon
- 2 carrots, (cut into slices)
- 3 garlic cloves, minced
- 1 yellow onion, chopped
- 1 rosemary bunch, torn
- A pinch of (ground) black pepper and salt
- 1 thyme bunch, torn

Cooking Instructions:

1. Preheat an oven to 425°F. Grease a baking dish with some cooking spray.
2. Add the chicken in the dish.
3. Mix the oil, rosemary, thyme, salt, pepper, and lemon juice in a bowl. Coat the chicken with it.

4. Add the carrots, potatoes and onion in the dish; bake for 60-70 minutes until cooked well.

5. Slice the chicken and serve warm.

Nutritional Values (Per Serving):

Calories 308, Fat 7g, Carbohydrates 16g, Fiber 3g, Protein 22g

Bean Chicken Chili

Recipe Time: 30 minutes

Serving Size: 4

Meal Type: Dinner

Diet Type: Gluten Free, Dairy Free, Soy Free, Nut Free

Ingredients:

- 1 pound chicken, ground
- 30 ounces canned black beans, drained and rinsed
- 28 ounces roasted tomatoes, chopped
- 3 cups butternut squash, cubed
- 1 cup yellow onion, chopped
- 1 ½ tablespoons olive oil
- 2 garlic cloves, minced
- 14 ounces chicken stock
- A pinch of (ground) black pepper and salt

Cooking Instructions:

1. In a skillet (you can also use a saucepan); heat the oil over medium stove flame.

2. Add the garlic, onion, chicken stir the mixture and cook while stirring for about 5-6 minutes until softened.

3. Add the beans, tomatoes, squash, stock, salt and pepper, toss the mix,

4. Simmer and cook for 12-15 minutes.

5. Add into serving bowls and serve warm.

Nutritional Values (Per Serving):

Calories 258, Fat 5g, Carbohydrates 10g, Fiber 4g, Protein 12g

Stuffed Pepper Delight

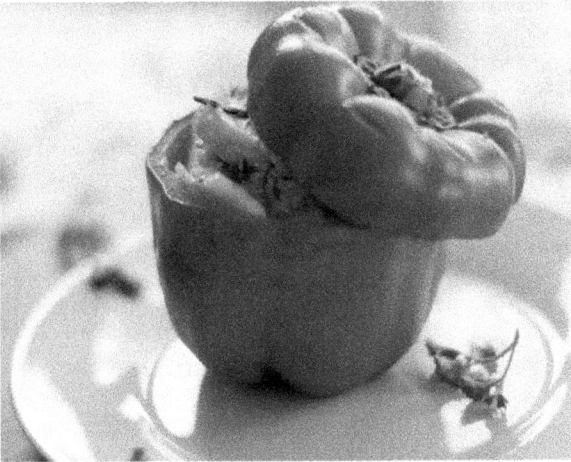

Recipe Time: 20 minutes

Serving Size: 3

Meal Type: Dinner

Diet Type: Gluten Free, Dairy Free, Soy Free, Nut Free

Ingredients:

- 1 small white onion, diced

- 2 garlic cloves, minced

- 1 (16-ounce) can diced tomatoes, drained

- 6 yellow, red or green bell peppers, tops and ribs removed, seeded

- 1 tablespoon avocado or coconut oil

- 1 pound ground turkey

- ½ teaspoon ground cumin

- ½ teaspoon paprika

- ½ teaspoon dried oregano

- ½ teaspoon salt

- Freshly ground black pepper

Cooking Instructions:

1. Preheat an oven to 400°F. Line a baking sheet with a foil.

2. Arrange the bell peppers on the sheet. Drizzle with some oil.

3. Bake for 20 minutes, or until softened.

4. In a skillet (you can also use a saucepan); heat the oil over medium stove flame.

5. Add the turkey and cook, while stirring, until becomes evenly brown for 4-5 minutes.

6. Add the onion and garlic; stir-cook for 8-10 minutes until softened.

7. Stir in the tomatoes, cumin, paprika, oregano, and salt, and season with pepper.

8. Fill the baked peppers with the meat mixture. Serve warm.

Nutritional Values (Per Serving):

Calories 193, Fat 9g, Carbohydrates 12g, Fiber 4g, Protein 14g

Orange Peas Chicken

Recipe Time: 20 minutes

Serving Size: 4

Meal Type: Dinner

Diet Type: Dairy Free, Nut Free

Ingredients:

- 1 red onion, (cut into slices)

- 2 cups sugar snap peas

- 2 garlic cloves, minced

- 1 ¼ pounds chicken breast, skinless, boneless and sliced

- 3 tablespoons coconut flour

- 2 tablespoons olive oil

- 2 tablespoons rice vinegar

- 1 tablespoon sesame seeds, toasted

- ½ cup teriyaki sauce

- 1 tablespoon sesame oil

- 2 oranges, peeled and sliced

- 1 tablespoon cilantro, chopped

Cooking Instructions:

1. In a bowl (medium size), mix the chicken, flour and toss well.

2. In a skillet (you can also use a saucepan); heat the oil over medium stove flame.

3. Add the chicken and cook, while stirring, until becomes evenly brown.

4. Add the garlic and the onion, stir-cook for 1-2 minutes.

5. Add the peas and cook for another 2 minutes.

6. Add the sauce, sesame oil, vinegar, sesame seeds, oranges and cilantro; stir-cook for 1-2 minutes.

7. Add the mix in serving plates and serve.

Nutritional Values (Per Serving):

Calories 287, Fat 3g, Carbohydrates 15g, Fiber 6g, Protein 13g

Herbed Broccoli Chicken

Recipe Time: 40-45 minutes

Serving Size: 4

Meal Type: Dinner

Diet Type: Gluten Free, Dairy Free, Soy Free, Nut Free

Ingredients:

- 2 teaspoons mustard
- 3 tablespoons olive oil
- 1 ½ tablespoons rosemary, chopped
- 2 tablespoons parsley, chopped
- 1 garlic clove, minced
- A pinch of (ground) black pepper and salt
- 1 broccoli head, florets separated
- 1 red onion, cut into wedges
- Juice of 1 lemon
- 4 chicken breasts, skin-on and bone-in
- ½ teaspoon red pepper, crushed

Cooking Instructions:

1. Preheat an oven to 425°F.
2. In a baking dish, mix the chicken with half of the oil, lemon juice, parsley, garlic, rosemary and mustard.
3. Coat well and bake for 30 minutes and divide between serving plates.

4. Line a baking sheet with a foil. Spread the broccoli florets, drizzle the rest of the oil over. Add the red onion and crushed pepper, toss gently.

5. Bake for 15 minutes, add next to the chicken and serve.

Nutritional Values (Per Serving):

Calories 268, Fat 13g, Carbohydrates 15g, Fiber 6g, Protein 27g

Pork, Beef & Lamb

Beef Yogurt Meatballs

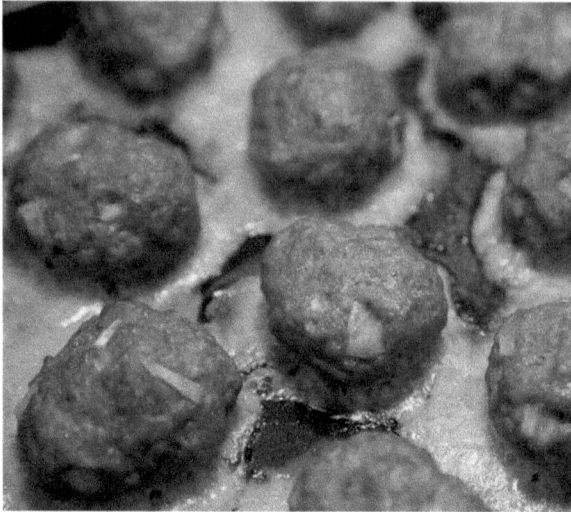

Recipe Time: 60 minutes

Serving Size: 4

Meal Type: Lunch

Diet Type: Gluten Free, Soy Free, Nut Free

Ingredients:

- 2/3 cup plain Greek yogurt
- 1 teaspoon honey
- 1 small sweet potato
- 3 garlic cloves, unpeeled
- 1 small onion, chopped finely
- 1 egg
- (ground) black pepper and salt, to taste, to taste
- ½ pound grass-fed ground beef

- 1 teaspoon ground coriander
- 1 teaspoon ground cumin
- ½ teaspoon cayenne pepper
- 1 tablespoon olive oil

Cooking Instructions:

1. Cook the potatoes to boiling water in a cooking pot for 25-30 minutes then drain.

2. Peel and mash them. Set aside in the large bowl.

3. In a skillet (you can also use a saucepan); heat the olive oil over medium stove flame.

4. Add the garlic, stir the mixture and cook while stirring for about 8-10 minutes until softened.

5. Add the cloves to the food processor or blender.

6. Add the yogurt, honey, salt, and black pepper.

7. Puree the mix until smooth and set aside.

8. Add the egg, ground beef, onion, salt, and spices with the potato bowl. Combine and prepare small meatballs out of this mixture.

9. Take a deep pan and heat oil in it.

10. Add the meatballs in batches and fry for 15-20 minutes until golden brown. Serve with the garlic yogurt.

Nutritional Values (Per Serving):

Calories 276, Fat 14g, Carbohydrates 28g, Fiber 3g, Protein 18g

Lamb Garlic Kebabs with Greens/Rice

Recipe Time: 20-25 minutes

Serving Size: 2-3

Meal Type: Lunch

Diet Type: Gluten Free, Dairy Free, Soy Free, Nut Free

Ingredients:

- 1 tablespoon dried oregano
- 2 teaspoons minced garlic
- 2 tablespoons olive oil
- 2 tablespoons apple cider vinegar
- ½ teaspoon sea salt
- 1 pound lamb shoulder, cut into 1-inch cubes

Cooking Instructions:

1. In a mixing bowl, combine the olive oil, cider vinegar, oregano, garlic, and sea salt.

2. Mix in the lamb. Cover and refrigerate it for 1-2 hour to marinate.

3. Preheat your broiler. Arrange a rack on higher side.

4. Take 8 wooden skewers, thread 4 or 5 pieces of lamb on each and arrange them on a baking sheet.

5. Broil for about 12-15 minutes total, turn in between, until browned evenly.

6. Serve with mixed greens or cooked rice (optional).

Nutritional Values (Per Serving):

Calories 426, Fat 26g, Carbohydrates 3g, Fiber 1g, Protein 54g

Cinnamon Pork Chops

Recipe Time: 35 minutes

Serving Size: 4

Meal Type: Lunch

Diet Type: Gluten Free, Dairy Free, Soy Free, Nut Free

Ingredients:

- 4 pork chops

- ½ teaspoon cinnamon powder

- ½ teaspoon sweet paprika

- A drizzle of olive oil

- A pinch of (ground) black pepper and salt

Cooking Instructions:

1. In a bowl (medium size), coat the pork chops with salt, pepper, oil, cinnamon and paprika.

2. Heat up a grill over medium-high flame.

3. Cook the pork chops for 10-15 minutes on each side, until cook well.

4. Serve with a side salad.

Nutritional Values (Per Serving):

Calories 248, Fat 6g, Carbohydrates 15g, Fiber 7g, Protein 17g

Mustard Lamb Lunch

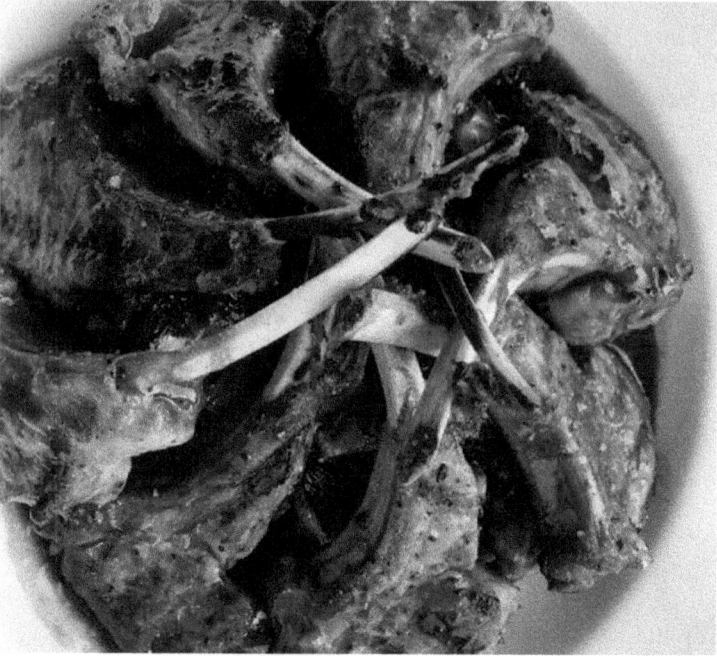

Recipe Time: 45 minutes

Serving Size: 4

Meal Type: Lunch

Diet Type: Gluten Free, Dairy Free, Soy Free, Nut Free

Ingredients:

- 2 (8-rib) lamb racks, patted dry

- ¼ cup Dijon mustard

- 2 tablespoons chopped fresh thyme

- 1 tablespoon chopped fresh rosemary

- Freshly ground black pepper and salt to taste

- 1 tablespoon olive oil

Cooking Instructions:

1. Preheat an oven to 425°F.

2. In a mixing bowl, stir together the mustard, thyme, and rosemary.

3. Coat the lamb racks with sea salt and pepper.

4. Place a large ovenproof skillet over medium-high cooking flame and heat the olive oil.

5. Add the lamb rack; stir-cook for about 2 minutes per side, turning once.

6. Take it off the heat and top with the mustard mix.

7. Bake for 30 minutes or until cooks well.

8. Remove the lamb racks and cut into pieces. Serve warm.

Nutritional Values (Per Serving):

Calories 413, Fat 24g, Carbohydrates 2g, Fiber 1g, Protein 52g

Bok Choy Steak Dinner

Recipe Time: 20 minutes

Serving Size: 4

Meal Type: Dinner

Diet Type: Gluten Free, Dairy Free, Soy Free, Nut Free

Ingredients:

- 2 teaspoons avocado oil

- 1 tablespoon sesame oil

- 2 garlic cloves, minced

- 12 ounces flank steak, cut into thin 2-inch strips

- ½ teaspoon salt

- ¼ teaspoon black pepper

- 4 heads baby bok choy, quartered lengthwise

- 1 tablespoon (shredded or grated) peeled fresh ginger

- 1 tablespoon coconut sugar or maple syrup

- 3 tablespoons coconut aminos

- 2 tablespoons rice vinegar

- ¼ teaspoon red pepper flakes (optional)

Cooking Instructions:

1. Season the with the salt and pepper.

2. In a skillet (you can also use a saucepan); heat the oil over medium stove flame.

3. Add the steak and cook, while stirring, until becomes evenly brown.

4. Transfer to a plate.

5. In the skillet, add the sesame oil and garlic. Stir-cook for 2-3 minutes.

6. Stir in the vinegar, ginger, coconut sugar, bok choy, coconut aminos, and red pepper flakes until well combined.

7. Cover and cook for 2 minutes.

8. Add the steak and toss gently; serve warm.

Nutritional Values (Per Serving):

Calories 246, Fat 13g, Carbohydrates 13g, Fiber 8g, Protein 21g

Apple Pork Raisins

Recipe Time: 40 minutes

Serving Size: 4

Meal Type: Dinner

Diet Type: Gluten Free, Dairy Free, Soy Free

Ingredients:

Salsa:

- ½ teaspoon (shredded or grated) fresh ginger
- 2 apples, peeled, cored, and diced
- 1 teaspoon olive oil
- ¼ cup finely chopped sweet onion
- ½ cup dried raisins
- Pinch sea salt

Chops:

- 4 (4-ounce) boneless center-cut pork chops, trimmed and patted dry
- Freshly ground black pepper and salt to taste
- 1 teaspoon garlic powder
- 1 teaspoon ground cinnamon
- 1 tablespoon olive oil

Cooking Instructions:

1. In a skillet (you can also use a saucepan); heat the oil over medium stove flame.

2. Add the onions, ginger, stir the mixture and cook while stirring for about 2-3 minutes until softened.

3. Stir in the apples and raisins. Sauté for about 4-5 minutes.

4. Season with sea salt and set it aside.

5. Coat the pork chops on both sides with the garlic powder, cinnamon, sea salt, and pepper.

6. In a skillet (you can also use a saucepan); heat the oil over medium stove flame.

7. Add the chops and cook, while stirring, until becomes evenly brown.

8. Serve the chops with the apple salsa.

Nutritional Values (Per Serving):

Calories 384, Fat 27g, Carbohydrates 11g, Fiber 2g, Protein 26g

Avocado Pineapple Pork

Recipe Time: 50 minutes

Serving Size: 4

Meal Type: Dinner

Diet Type: Gluten Free, Dairy Free, Soy Free, Nut Free

Ingredients:

- 1 teaspoon cumin
- 8 ounces canned pineapple, crushed
- 1 tablespoon olive oil
- 1 pound pork, ground
- 1 teaspoon chili powder
- 1 teaspoon garlic powder
- (ground) black pepper and salt to taste
- 1 mango, chopped
- Juice of 1 lime
- 2 avocados, pitted, peeled and chopped
- ¼ cup cilantro, chopped

Cooking Instructions:

1. In a skillet (you can also use a saucepan); heat the oil over medium stove flame.

2. Add the pork and cook, while stirring, until becomes evenly brown.

3. Add the garlic, cumin, chili powder, salt and pepper, stir-cook for 7-8 minutes.

4. Add the pineapple, mango, avocados, lime juice, cilantro, salt and pepper; stir-cook for 5-6 minutes.

5. Divide between serving plates and serve.

Nutritional Values (Per Serving):

Calories 238, Fat 6g, Carbohydrates 12g, Fiber 7g, Protein 17g

Herbed Tomato Chops

Recipe Time: 65-70 minutes

Serving Size: 4

Meal Type: Dinner

Diet Type: Gluten Free, Dairy Free, Soy Free, Nut Free

Ingredients:

- 28 ounces canned tomatoes, chopped

- ¼ cup chicken stock

- 1 cup tomato sauce

- ¼ cup balsamic vinegar

- 2 tablespoons olive oil

- 4 pork chops

- A pinch of (ground) black pepper and salt

- 2 garlic cloves, minced

- 1 yellow onion, chopped

- 1 tablespoon herbs de Provence

- 2 tablespoons parsley, chopped

- 1 tablespoon basil, chopped

Cooking Instructions:

1. In a skillet (you can also use a saucepan); heat the oil over medium stove flame.

2. Add the pork, pepper, salt and cook, while stirring, until becomes evenly brown.

3. Transfer to a serving plate.

4. In a skillet (you can also use a saucepan); heat the oil over medium stove flame.

5. Add the onions, garlic, stir the mixture and cook while stirring for about 8-10 minutes until softened.

6. Add the tomatoes, stock, tomato sauce, vinegar, herbs and parsley, stir-cook for 8-10 minutes.

7. Add the pork and basil, stir, cook for 4-5 minutes more. Add the mix between plates and serve.

Nutritional Values (Per Serving):

Calories 208, Fat 6g, Carbohydrates 9g, Fiber 5g, Protein 18g

Garlic Basil Pork Chops

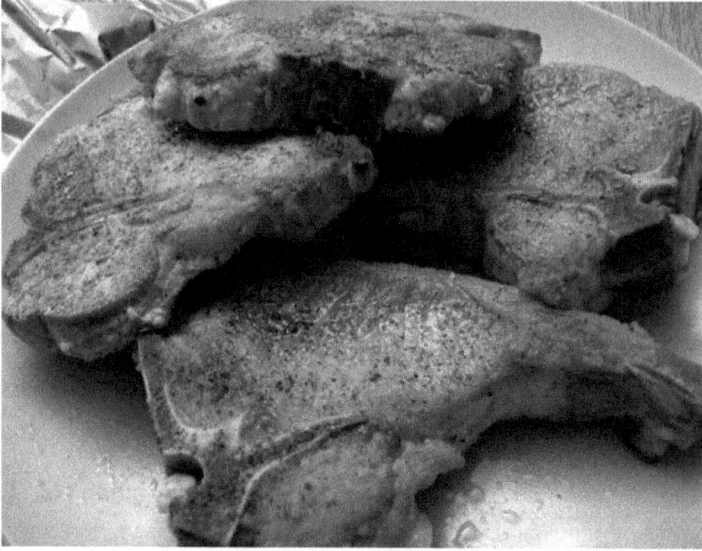

Recipe Time: 20 minutes

Serving Size: 4

Meal Type: Dinner

Diet Type: Gluten Free, Dairy Free, Soy Free, Nut Free

Ingredients:

- 1 cup basil, minced

- 2 tablespoons lemon juice

- 4 pork loin chops

- 2 tablespoons garlic, minced

- 2 tablespoons olive oil

- A pinch of (ground) black pepper and salt

Cooking Instructions:

1. In a bowl (medium size), mix the garlic, oil, basil, lemon juice, salt and pepper. Combine well.

2. Add pork chops and toss well.

3. Place the chops over the preheated grill; cook them for 6 minutes on each side.

4. Add in serving plates and serve warm.

Nutritional Values (Per Serving):

Calories 314, Fat 6g, Carbohydrates 19g, Fiber 6g, Protein 23g

Nutty Pork Steak

Recipe Time: 15 minutes

Serving Size: 4

Meal Type: Dinner

Diet Type: Gluten Free, Dairy Free, Soy Free

Ingredients:

- ¼ cup basil, chopped

- 1 tablespoons garlic, minced

- ¼ cup balsamic vinegar

- 1 pound pork steaks

- 2 tablespoons olive oil

- (ground) black pepper and salt to taste

- 1 teaspoon onion powder

For the pesto:

- ¼ cup olive oil

- ¼ cup pine nuts

- ½ cup bell peppers, roasted

- ½ cup basil, chopped

- 1 garlic clove

- (ground) black pepper and salt to taste

Cooking Instructions:

1. In a bowl (medium size), season the steaks with vinegar, 2 tablespoons oil, basil, garlic, onion, salt and pepper. Add in the fridge for 3-4 hours.

2. Heat your grill over medium-high cooking flame, add the steaks, cook for 4 minutes each side.

3. In your food processor or blender, add the basil with roasted peppers, pine nuts, ¼ cup olive oil, garlic, salt and pepper. Blend to make a smooth mix.

Serve the steaks with the pesto on top.

Nutritional Values (Per Serving):

Calories 276, Fat 7g, Carbohydrates 18g, Fiber 5g, Protein 21g

Beef Bread-Less Meatloaf

Recipe Time: 60 minutes

Serving Size: 4

Meal Type: Dinner

Diet Type: Gluten Free, Dairy Free, Soy Free, Nut Free

Ingredients:

- 1 egg
- 1½ pounds lean ground beef
- ½ cup almond flour
- ½ cup chopped sweet onion
- 1 tablespoon chopped fresh basil
- 1 tablespoon chopped fresh parsley
- 1 teaspoon (shredded or grated) fresh horseradish
- ⅛ teaspoon sea salt

Cooking Instructions:

1. Preheat an oven to 350°F. Grease a loaf pan with some cooking spray.

2. In a mixing bowl, combine the beef, almond flour, onion, egg, basil, parsley, horseradish, and sea salt.

3. Add the meat mixture into the loaf pan.

4. Bake for about 55-60 minutes until cooked through.

5. Remove the pan and serve warm.

Nutritional Values (Per Serving):

Calories 412, Fat 17g, Carbohydrates 5g, Fiber 2g, Protein 53g

Zucchini Jalapeno Pork Meal

Recipe Time: 30 minutes

Serving Size: 4

Meal Type: Dinner

Diet Type: Gluten Free, Dairy Free, Soy Free, Nut Free

Ingredients:

- 3 tablespoons lime juice

- 1 tablespoon olive oil

- 1 jalapeno, halved and seeded

- 3 tomatoes, halved

- 1 red onion, halved

- 4 pork steaks

- 2 zucchinis, (cut into slices)

- ½ cup cilantro, chopped

- 1 garlic clove, minced

- A pinch of(ground) black pepper and salt

Cooking Instructions:

1. Preheat an oven to 475°F. Grease a roasting pan with some cooking spray.

2. Add the tomatoes, zucchini, jalapeno and onion in the pan, and bake for 10 minutes.

3. In a bowl (medium size), mix the olive oil with garlic, cilantro, lime juice, black pepper and salt, whisk.

4. Add to the pan, toss well and divide between serving plates.

5. In a skillet (you can also use a saucepan); coat with some cooking spray. .

6. Add the steak, salt, pepper and cook, while stirring, until becomes evenly brown.

7. Add it with the veggies and serve.

Nutritional Values (Per Serving):

Calories 215, Fat9 g, Carbohydrates 10g, Fiber 3g, Protein 24g

Berry Chops Dinner

Recipe Time: 25 minutes

Serving Size: 4

Meal Type: Dinner

Diet Type: Gluten Free, Dairy Free, Soy Free, Nut Free

Ingredients:

- 2 pounds pork chops
- ½ teaspoon thyme, dried
- 2 tablespoons water
- 1 teaspoon cinnamon powder
- (ground) black pepper and salt to taste
- 12 ounces blackberries
- ½ cup balsamic vinegar

Cooking Instructions:

1. Season pork chops with salt, pepper, cinnamon and thyme.

2. Heat up a cooking pot; add the blackberries and heat over medium heat.

3. Add the vinegar, water, salt and pepper, stir the mix.

4. Simmer for 3-5 minutes and take it off the heat.

5. Brush the pork chops with half of the blueberry mix.

6. Preheat your grill and grill the chops over medium heat for 6 minutes on each side.

7. Divide the pork chops between serving plates; top with the rest of the blackberry sauce. Serve warm.

Nutritional Values (Per Serving):

Calories 286, Fat 6g, Carbohydrates 11g, Fiber 6g, Protein 22g

Cauliflower Lamb Meal

Recipe Time: 25 minutes

Serving Size: 4

Meal Type: Dinner

Diet Type: Gluten Free, Soy Free, Nut Free

Ingredients:

Mash:

- 1 large head cauliflower, cut into florets

- ½ teaspoon garlic powder

- ½ teaspoon salt

- Dash cayenne pepper

Lamb:

- 2 (8-ounce) grass-fed lamb fillets

- 2 tablespoons avocado oil

- 1 teaspoon dried rosemary

- 1 teaspoon salt

- ½ teaspoon freshly ground black pepper

Cooking Instructions:

1. In a cooking (you can also use a saucepan); add the cauliflower and water to cover it.

2. Heat it over medium stove flame. Boil and cook for 10 minutes. Drain water and transfer the cauliflower to a food processor (or blender).

3. Add the ghee, garlic powder, salt, and cayenne pepper. Blend to a smooth consistency.

4. Season the lamb with the salt and pepper.

5. In a skillet (you can also use a saucepan); heat the oil over medium stove flame.

6. Add the lamb, rosemary and cook, while stirring, until becomes evenly brown for 8-10 minutes.

7. Slice the lamb into coins and serve with the cauliflower mash.

Nutritional Values (Per Serving):

Calories 294, Fat 17g, Carbohydrates 11g, Fiber 3g, Protein 36g

Grilled Mint Chops

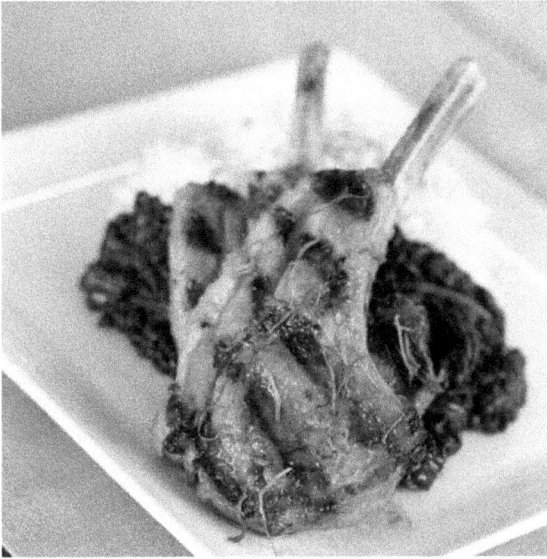

Recipe Time: 20 minutes

Serving Size: 4

Meal Type: Dinner

Diet Type: Gluten Free, Dairy Free, Soy Free, Nut Free

Ingredients:

- 8 lamb chops

- ¼ cup white vinegar

- ½ cup olive oil

- 1 cup mint leaves

- ¼ cup parsley leaves

- 2 garlic cloves, minced

- (ground) black pepper and salt to the taste

- ¼ teaspoon red pepper flakes

Cooking Instructions:

1. In a blender, add the mint, parsley, vinegar, oil, garlic, salt, pepper and pepper flakes, blend to make a smooth mix.

2. Coat the pork chops with this mix and marinate for 30-60 minutes.

3. Place the chops on the preheated grill; cook over medium-high heat for 6-7 minutes on each side.

4. Add in serving plates and serve with the leftover the mint sauce.

Nutritional Values (Per Serving):

Calories 256, Fat 8g, Carbohydrates 9g, Fiber 1g, Protein 24g

Sprouts Pork Chops

Recipe Time: 30 minutes

Serving Size: 4

Meal Type: Dinner

Diet Type: Gluten Free, Dairy Free, Soy Free, Nut Free

Ingredients:

- 1 pound pork chops, boneless
- 1 teaspoon mustard
- ½ tablespoon balsamic vinegar
- ¼ cup onion, chopped
- A pinch of (ground) black pepper and salt
- 1 ½ tablespoons olive oil
- 1 ¼ cup Brussels sprouts, halved
- 2/3 cup chicken stock
- ¼ cup applesauce, unsweetened
- 2 garlic cloves, minced
- 1 tablespoon rosemary, chopped
- 1 tablespoon sage, chopped

Cooking Instructions:

1. In a skillet (you can also use a saucepan); heat half the oil over medium stove flame.

2. Add the chops, salt, pepper, and cook, while stirring, until becomes evenly brown.

3. Transfer to a plate.

4. In the pan, heat rest of the oil, add the stock, mustard, vinegar, onion, applesauce, garlic, rosemary and sage.

5. Stir well and simmer the mix; cook for 5-6 minutes.

6. Add the sprouts, toss and cook for 4-5 minutes.

7. Add the pork chops, toss, cook mixture for a 2-3 minutes. Add in serving plates and serve.

Nutritional Values (Per Serving):

Calories 254, Fat 6g, Carbohydrates 11g, Fiber 7g, Protein 19g

Fish & Seafood

Shrimp Mushroom Squash

Recipe Time: 20 minutes

Serving Size: 4

Meal Type: Lunch

Diet Type: Gluten Free, Dairy Free, Soy Free, Nut Free

Ingredients:

- 2 tablespoons hemp seeds

- 2 tablespoons olive oil

- 1 pound shrimp, peeled and deveined

- ¼ cup coconut aminos

- 2 tablespoons raw honey

- 2 teaspoons sesame oil

- 1 yellow onion, chopped

- 4 ounces shiitake mushrooms, (cut into slices)

- 2 garlic cloves, minced

- 1 red bell pepper, (cut into slices)

- 1 yellow squash, peeled and cubed

- 2 cups chard, chopped

Cooking Instructions:

1. In a bowl (medium size), mix the aminos, honey, sesame oil and hemp seeds.

2. In a skillet (you can also use a saucepan); heat the oil over medium stove flame.

3. Add the onions, stir the mixture and cook while stirring for about 2-3 minutes until softened.

4. Add the bell pepper, squash, mushrooms and garlic, stir-cook for 5 minutes.

5. Add the shrimp and aminos mix; stir-cook for 4 minutes more.

6. Add the chard, toss; add into serving bowls and serve.

Nutritional Values (Per Serving):

Calories 236, Fat 8g, Carbohydrates 11g, Fiber 5g, Protein 9g

Spinach Sea Bass Lunch

Recipe Time: 30 minutes

Serving Size: 2

Meal Type: Lunch

Diet Type: Gluten Free, Dairy Free, Soy Free, Nut Free

Ingredients:

- 2 sea bass fillets, boneless
- 2 shallots, chopped
- Juice of ½ lemon
- 1 garlic clove, minced
- 5 cherry tomatoes, halved
- 1 tablespoon parsley, chopped
- 1 tablespoon olive oil
- 8 ounces baby spinach

Cooking Instructions:

1. Preheat an oven to 450°F. Grease a baking dish with some cooking spray.
2. Add the fish, tomatoes, parsley and garlic, drizzle the lemon juice.
3. Cover the dish and bake for 12-15 minutes and add in serving plates.
4. In a skillet (you can also use a saucepan); heat the oil over medium stove flame.
5. Add the shallots, stir the mixture and cook while stirring for about 1-2 minutes until softened.

6. Add the spinach, stir, cook for 4-5 minutes more. Add with the fish and serve warm.

Nutritional Values (Per Serving):

Calories 218, Fat 3g, Carbohydrates 11g, Fiber 6g, Protein 24g

Garlic Cod Meal

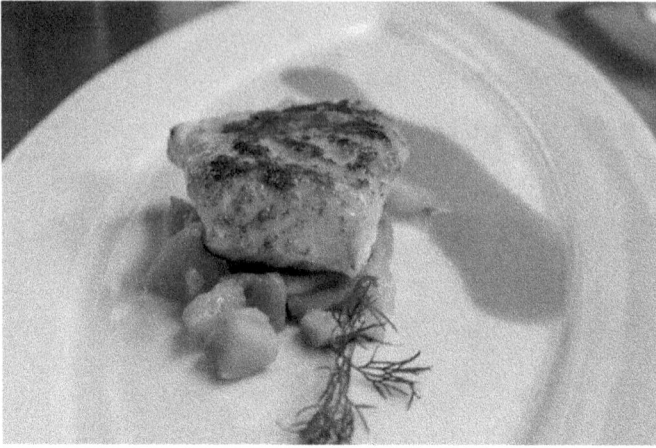

Recipe Time: 35 minutes

Serving Size: 4

Meal Type: Lunch

Diet Type: Gluten Free, Dairy Free, Soy Free, Nut Free

Ingredients:

- 2 tablespoons olive oil
- 2 tablespoons tarragon, chopped
- ¼ cup parsley, chopped
- 4 cod fillets, skinless
- 3 garlic cloves, minced
- 1 yellow onion, chopped
- (ground) black pepper and salt to the taste

- Juice of 1 lemon
- 1 lemon, (cut into slices)
- 1 tablespoon thyme, chopped
- 4 cups water

Cooking Instructions:

1. In a skillet (you can also use a saucepan); heat the oil over medium stove flame.

2. Add the onions, garlic, stir the mixture and cook while stirring for about 2-3 minutes until softened.

3. Add the salt, pepper, tarragon, parsley, thyme, water, lemon juice and lemon slices.

4. Boil the mix; add the cod, cook for 12-15 minutes, drain the liquid.

5. Serve with a side salad.

Nutritional Values (Per Serving):

Calories 181, Fat 3g, Carbohydrates 9g, Fiber 4g, Protein 12g

Cod Cucumber Delight

Recipe Time: 25 minutes

Serving Size: 4

Meal Type: Lunch

Diet Type: Gluten Free, Dairy Free, Soy Free, Nut Free

Ingredients:

- 1 tablespoon capers, drained

- 4 tablespoons + 1 teaspoon olive oil

- 4 cod fillets, skinless and boneless

- 2 tablespoons mustard

- 1 tablespoon tarragon, chopped

- (ground) black pepper and salt to the taste

- 2 cups lettuce leaves, torn

- 1 small red onion, (cut into slices)

- 1 small cucumber, (cut into slices)

- 2 tablespoons lemon juice

- 2 tablespoons water

Cooking Instructions:

1. In a bowl (medium size), mix the mustard with 2 tablespoons olive oil, tarragon, capers and water, whisk well and set aside.

2. In a skillet (you can also use a saucepan); heat 1 teaspoon oil over medium stove flame.

3. Add the fish, pepper, salt and cook, while stirring, until cooks well and turn softened on both sides.

4. In a bowl (medium size), mix the cucumber, onion, lettuce, lemon juice, 2 tablespoons olive oil, salt and pepper.

5. Arrange the cod in serving plates, top with the tarragon sauce.

6. Serve with the cucumber salad.

Nutritional Values (Per Serving):

Calories 284, Fat 8g, Carbohydrates 9g, Fiber 1g, Protein 14g

Salmon Greens

Recipe Time: 30 minutes

Serving Size: 6

Meal Type: Lunch

Diet Type: Gluten Free, Dairy Free, Soy Free, Nut Free

Ingredients:

- 4 salmon fillets, boneless and skin-on

- 15 ounces Brussels sprouts, halved

- 15 ounces baby potatoes, halved

- 1 bunch asparagus, halved and trimmed

- 1 small red onion, cubed

- 3 tablespoons balsamic vinegar

- 1 tablespoon mustard

- 2 tablespoons olive oil

- 1 cup cherry tomatoes, halved

- 1 garlic clove, minced

- 1 teaspoon thyme, chopped

- A pinch of (ground) black pepper and salt

Cooking Instructions:

1. Preheat an oven to 450°F. Grease a baking dish with some cooking spray.

2. Spread the potatoes on the sheet.

3. Add the asparagus, sprouts, onion, tomatoes, vinegar, garlic, salt, pepper, thyme and oil, toss the mix.

4. Bake for 8-10 minutes.

5. Add the salmon, season with salt and pepper, bake for 10 minutes more,

6. Add the mix in serving plates and serve.

Nutritional Values (Per Serving):

Calories 253, Fat 10g, Carbohydrates 13g, Fiber 6g, Protein 9g

Oregano Lettuce Shrimp

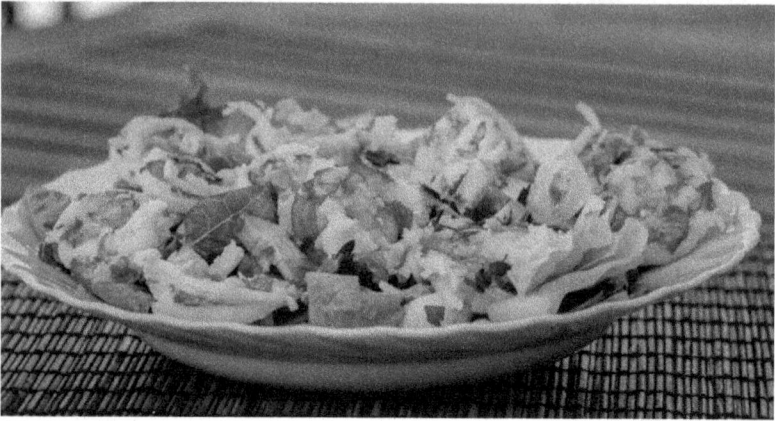

Recipe Time: 25 minutes

Serving Size: 4

Meal Type: Lunch

Diet Type: Gluten Free, Dairy Free, Soy Free, Nut Free

Ingredients:

- 3 tablespoons dill, chopped

- 1 tablespoon oregano, chopped

- 2 garlic cloves, chopped

- 1 pound shrimp, deveined and peeled

- 2 teaspoons olive oil

- 6 tablespoons lemon juice

- (ground) black pepper and salt to taste

- 2 cucumbers, (cut into slices)

- 1 red onion, (cut into slices)

- ¾ cup coconut cream

- ½ pounds cherry tomatoes

- 8 lettuce leaves

Cooking Instructions:

1. In a bowl (medium size), combine the shrimp, 1 tablespoon oregano, 2 tablespoons lemon juice, 1 tablespoon dill, and 1 teaspoon oil. Set aside for 10 minutes.

2. In another bowl, mix 1 tablespoon dill, half of the garlic, ¼ cup coconut cream, 2 tablespoons lemon juice, cucumber, salt and pepper. Combine well.

3. In another bowl, mix rest of the lemon juice, ½ cup cream, the rest of the garlic and the rest of the dill.

4. In a bowl (medium size), mix the tomatoes with onion and 1 teaspoon olive oil.

5. Heat a grill over medium-high heat, grill tomato mix and shrimp mix for 5 minutes,

6. Add them in serving plates, add the cucumber salad, lettuce leaves and other ingredients on top.

Nutritional Values (Per Serving):

Calories 268, Fat 5g, Carbohydrates 12g, Fiber 6g, Protein 11g

Mexican Pepper Salmon

Recipe Time: 25 minutes

Serving Size: 4

Meal Type: Lunch

Diet Type: Gluten Free, Dairy Free, Soy Free, Nut Free

Ingredients:

- 1 garlic clove, minced

- 1 teaspoon sweet paprika

- 4 medium salmon fillets, boneless

- 2 teaspoons olive oil

- 4 teaspoons lemon juice

- A pinch of (ground) black pepper and salt

For the salsa:

- 4 teaspoons oregano, chopped

- 1 small habanero pepper, chopped

- ¼ cup green onions, chopped

- 1 cup red bell pepper, chopped

- 1 garlic clove, minced

- ¼ cup lemon juice

Cooking Instructions:

1. In a bowl (medium size), combine the green onion, ¼ cup lemon juice, bell pepper, habanero, 1 garlic clove, oregano, black pepper and salt.

2. In a another bowl, mix the paprika, 4 teaspoons lemon juice, olive oil, and 1 garlic clove.

3. Stir the mix, cot the fish with this mix; set aside for 10 minutes.

4. Add the fish on the preheated grill over medium-high heat setting.

5. Season the fish with black pepper and salt, cook for 5 minutes on each side.

6. Add between serving plates, top with the salsa and serve.

Nutritional Values (Per Serving):

Calories 198, Fat 4g, Carbohydrates 14g, Fiber 2g, Protein 8g

Fish Curry Dinner

Recipe Time: 30 minutes

Serving Size: 4

Meal Type: Dinner

Diet Type: Gluten Free, Dairy Free, Soy Free, Nut Free

Ingredients:

- 1 tablespoon red curry paste

- 1½ cups chicken broth

- 1 (14-ounce) can coconut milk

- 1 tablespoon avocado oil

- ½ cup diced white onion

- 2 garlic cloves, minced

- ½ teaspoon coconut sugar

- 1 teaspoon salt

- ½ teaspoon ground black pepper

- 4 (4-ounce) halibut fillets

Cooking Instructions:

1. In a skillet (you can also use a saucepan); heat the oil over medium stove flame.

2. Add the onions, garlic, stir the mixture and cook while stirring for about 2-3 minutes until softened.

3. Stir in the paste. Add the broth, coconut milk, coconut sugar, salt, and pepper; combine well.

4. Reduce the heat to low and simmer for 8-10 minutes.

5. Add the fillets; cover and cook for 8-10 minutes, until flakes easily.

6. Serve the fillets with the curried broth.

Nutritional Values (Per Serving):

Calories 326, Fat 21g, Carbohydrates 13g, Fiber 2g, Protein 27g

Salmon Broccoli Bowl

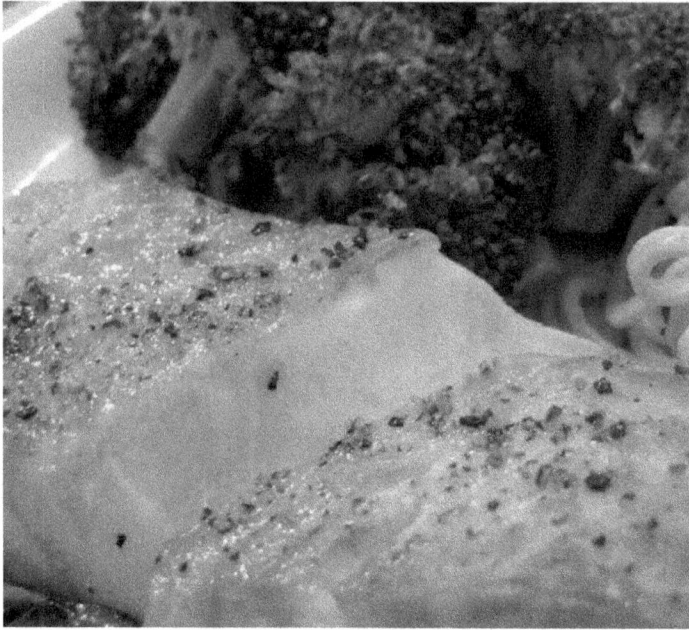

Recipe Time: 20 minutes

Serving Size: 4

Meal Type: Lunch

Diet Type: Gluten Free, Dairy Free, Soy Free, Nut Free

Ingredients:

- 3 tablespoons avocado oil

- 2 garlic cloves, minced

- 1 broccoli head, separate florets

- 1 ½ pounds salmon fillets, boneless

- A pinch of (ground) black pepper and salt

- Juice of ½ lemon

Cooking Instructions:

1. Preheat an oven to 450°F. Line a baking sheet with a foil.

2. Spread the broccoli; add the salmon, oil, garlic, salt, pepper and the lemon juice, toss gently.

3. Bake for 15 minutes.

4. Divide in serving plates and serve warm.

Nutritional Values (Per Serving):

Calories 207, Fat 6g, Carbohydrates 14g, Fiber 6g, Protein 9g

Fennel Baked Cod

Recipe Time: 25 minutes

Serving Size: 4

Meal Type: Dinner

Diet Type: Gluten Free, Dairy Free, Soy Free, Nut Free

Ingredients:

- 3 sun-dried tomatoes, chopped
- 1 small red onion, (cut into slices)
- ½ fennel bulb,(cut into slices)
- 2 cod fillets, boneless
- 1 garlic cloves, minced
- 1 teaspoon olive oil
- Black pepper to the taste
- 4 black olives, pitted and sliced
- 2 rosemary springs
- ¼ teaspoon red pepper flakes

Cooking Instructions:

1. Preheat an oven to 400°F. Grease a baking dish with some cooking spray.

2. Add the cod, garlic, black pepper, tomatoes, onion, fennel, olives, rosemary and pepper flakes; mix gently.

3.   Bake for 14-15 minutes.

4.   Divide the fish mix between plates and serve.

Nutritional Values (Per Serving):

Calories 255, Fat 4g, Carbohydrates 11g, Fiber 6g, Protein 16g

Beet Haddock Dinner

Recipe Time: 40-45 minutes

Serving Size: 4

Meal Type: Dinner

Diet Type: Gluten Free, Dairy Free, Soy Free, Nut Free

Ingredients:

- 2 tablespoons olive oil
- 2 tablespoons apple cider vinegar
- 1 teaspoon chopped fresh thyme
- 8 beets, peeled and cut into small chunks
- 2 shallots, (cut into slices)
- 1 teaspoon minced garlic
- Pinch sea salt to taste
- 4 (5-ounce) haddock fillets, patted dry

Cooking Instructions:

1. Preheat an oven to 400°F. Grease a baking dish with some cooking spray.
2. In a bowl (medium size), mix the beets, shallots, garlic, and 1 tablespoon olive oil.
3. Add the beet mixture in the baking dish.
4. Bake for about 25-30 minutes, or until the vegetables are caramelized.
5. Remove from oven and stir in the cider vinegar, thyme, and sea salt.
6. In a skillet (you can also use a saucepan); heat the remaining oil over medium stove flame.

7. Add the fish, stir the mixture and cook while stirring for 12-15 minutes until cooks well.

8. Flake the fish and serve with roasted beets.

Nutritional Values (Per Serving):

Calories 324, Fat 8g, Carbohydrates 22g, Fiber 3g, Protein 37g

Honey Scallops

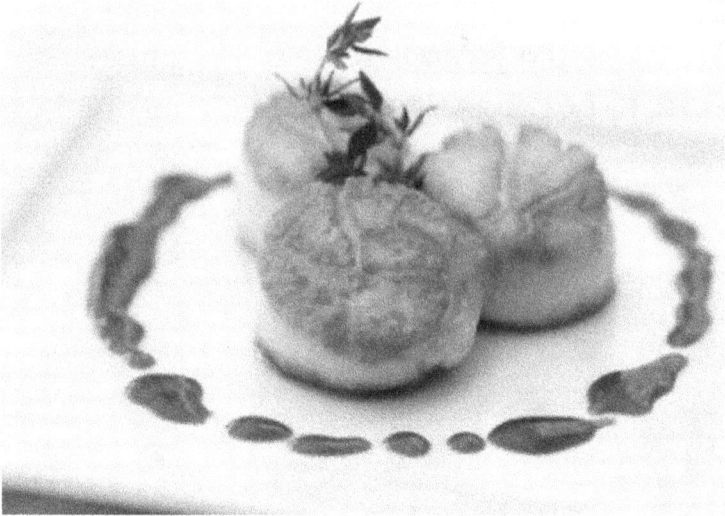

Recipe Time: 25 minutes

Serving Size: 4

Meal Type: Dinner

Diet Type: Gluten Free, Dairy Free, Soy Free, Nut Free

Ingredients:

- 1 pound large scallops, rinsed
- Dash of ground black pepper and salt to taste
- 3 tablespoons coconut aminos
- 2 garlic cloves, minced

- 2 tablespoons avocado oil

- ¼ cup raw honey

- 1 tablespoon apple cider vinegar

Cooking Instructions:

1. Sprinkle the scallops with the salt and pepper.

2. In a skillet (you can also use a saucepan); heat the oil over medium stove flame.

3. Add the scallops, stir the mixture and cook while stirring for about 2-3 minutes until softened and golden.

4. Transfer to a plate, and set aside.

5. In the same skillet or pan, heat the honey, coconut aminos, garlic, and vinegar.

6. Cook for 6-7 minutes; add the scallops and coat well. Serve warm.

Nutritional Values (Per Serving):

Calories 346, Fat 17g, Carbohydrates 27g, Fiber 2g, Protein 21g

Kale Cod Secret

Recipe Time: 30 minutes

Serving Size: 4

Meal Type: Dinner

Diet Type: Gluten Free, Dairy Free, Soy Free, Nut Free

Ingredients:

- 4 cod fillets, skinless and boneless

- 1 tablespoon ginger, (shredded or grated)

- 4 teaspoons lemon zest

- A pinch of (ground) black pepper and salt

- 3 leeks, chopped

- 2 cups veggie stock

- 2 tablespoons lemon juice

- 2 tablespoons olive oil

- 1 pound kale, chopped

- ½ teaspoon sesame oil

Cooking Instructions:

1. In a bowl (medium size), mix the zest with salt and pepper. Coat the fish with this mix.

2. In a skillet (you can also use a saucepan); heat the leeks, ginger and lemon juice over medium stove flame.

3. Heat for a few minutes; add the fish fillets.

4. Cover and cook for 8-10 minutes, transfer it to a plate.

5. Strain the liquid and reserve the leeks. Add the fish in serving plates.

6. In a skillet (you can also use a saucepan); heat the oil over medium stove flame.

7. Add the kale, stir the mixture and cook while stirring for about 3-4 minutes until softened.

8. Add the soup liquid and cook for 4-5 minutes more.

9. Add the reserved leeks; cook for 2 minutes.

10. Divide into fish bowls, drizzle the sesame oil all over and serve.

Nutritional Values (Per Serving):

Calories 238, Fat 3g, Carbohydrates 12g, Fiber 4g, Protein 16g

Scrumptious Coconut Shrimps

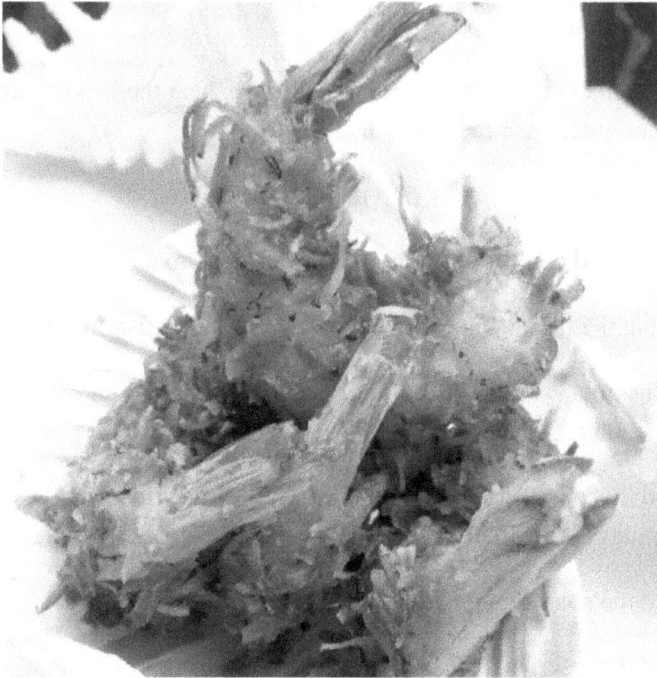

Recipe Time: 15-20 minutes

Serving Size: 4

Meal Type: Dinner

Diet Type: Gluten Free, Dairy Free, Soy Free, Nut Free

Ingredients:

- 2 eggs

- 1 cup dried shredded coconut, unsweetened

- ¼ teaspoon paprika

- Dash cayenne pepper

- ¼ cup coconut flour

- ½ teaspoon salt

- Dash freshly ground black pepper

- ¼ cup coconut oil

- 1 pound raw shrimp, peeled and deveined

Cooking Instructions:

1. In a bowl, whisk the eggs.

2. In another bowl, mix the coconut, flour, salt, paprika, cayenne pepper, and black pepper.

3. Coat the shrimp into the egg mixture, and then into the coconut mix.

4. In a skillet (you can also use a saucepan); heat the oil over medium stove flame.

5. Add the shrimps and cook for 2-3 minutes per side. Serve warm.

Nutritional Values (Per Serving):

Calories 246, Fat 18g, Carbohydrates 8g, Fiber 3g, Protein 19g

Herbed Mussels Treat

Recipe Time: 30 minutes

Serving Size: 4

Meal Type: Dinner

Diet Type: Gluten Free, Dairy Free, Soy Free, Nut Free

Ingredients:

- 1 tablespoon olive oil
- 2 teaspoons minced garlic
- 1 cup coconut milk
- ½ cup chicken bone broth
- 2 teaspoons chopped fresh thyme
- 1 teaspoon chopped fresh oregano
- 1½ pounds mussels, scrubbed and debearded
- 1 scallion, sliced white and green parts

Cooking Instructions:

1. In a skillet (you can also use a saucepan); heat the oil over medium stove flame.

2. Add the garlic, stir the mixture and cook while stirring for about 2-3 minutes until softened.

3. Add the coconut milk, broth, thyme, and oregano.

4. Boil the mix and add the mussels. Cover and cook for about 8 minutes, or until the shells opened up.

5. Remove any unopened shells and add in the scallion; serve warm.

Nutritional Values (Per Serving):

Calories 318, Fat 21g, Carbohydrates 12g, Fiber 2g, Protein 23g

Coconut Chili Salmon

Recipe Time: 25 minutes

Serving Size: 6

Meal Type: Dinner

Diet Type: Gluten Free, Dairy Free, Soy Free, Nut Free

Ingredients:

- 1 ¼ cups coconut, shredded

- 2 tablespoons olive oil

- ¼ cup water

- 1 pound salmon, cubed

- 1/3 cup coconut flour

- A pinch of (ground) black pepper and salt

- 1 egg

- 4 red chilies, chopped

- 3 garlic cloves, minced

- ¼ cup balsamic vinegar

- ½ cup raw honey

Cooking Instructions:

1. In a bowl (medium size), mix the flour with a pinch of salt.

2. In another bowl, whisk the egg and black pepper.

3. Add the shredded coconut in another bowl.

4. Coat the salmon cubes in flour, egg and coconut mix one by one.

5. In a skillet (you can also use a saucepan); heat the oil over medium stove flame.

6. Add the salmon, stir-fry them for 2-3 minutes on each side. Place in serving plates.

7. Heat water over medium-high heat in the pan, add the chilies, cloves, vinegar and honey, stir gently.

8. Boil the mix and simmer for 4 minutes; top over the salmon and serve.

Nutritional Values (Per Serving):

Calories 218, Fat 5g, Carbohydrates 14g, Fiber 2g, Protein 17g

Vegan & Vegetarian

Cauliflower Coconut Curry

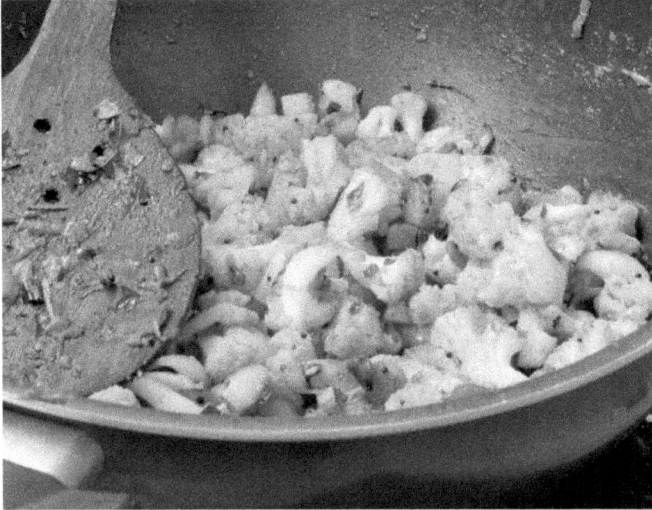

Recipe Time: 55 minutes

Serving Size: 4

Meal Type: Lunch

Diet Type: Gluten Free, Dairy Free, Soy Free, Nut Free, Vegan, Vegetarian

Ingredients:

- 3 cups vegetable stock

- 3 pounds cauliflower, florets separated

- 2 garlic cloves, minced

- 2 carrots, chopped

- 1 yellow onion, chopped

- 1 tablespoon coconut oil

- A pinch of (ground) black pepper and salt

- ½ cup coconut milk

- A pinch of nutmeg

- A pinch of cayenne pepper

- A handful parsley, chopped

Cooking Instructions:

1. In a skillet (you can also use a saucepan); heat the oil over medium stove flame.

2. Add the onions, carrots, garlic, stir the mixture and cook while stirring for about 4-5 minutes until softened.

3. Add the cauliflower and stock. Boil the mix and reduce heat; cover, cook for 40-45 minutes.

4. Add the mix to a blender, add the milk, salt and pepper.

5. Blend well and add into the bowls; sprinkle nutmeg, cayenne and parsley. Serve warm.

Nutritional Values (Per Serving):

Calories 234, Fat 2g, Carbohydrates 11g, Fiber 5g, Protein 7g

Pomegranate Kale Salad

Recipe Time: 15 minutes

Serving Size: 4

Meal Type: Lunch

Diet Type: Gluten Free, Dairy Free, Soy Free, Nut Free, Vegan, Vegetarian

Ingredients:

- ¼ cup shelled sunflower seeds
- 2 tablespoons lemon juice
- 2 bunches kale, stemmed and chopped
- 3 scallions, (cut into slices)
- 1 avocado, diced
- 3 tablespoons extra-virgin olive oil
- ½ teaspoon salt
- Freshly ground black pepper
- ¼ cup pomegranate pips

Cooking Instructions:

1. In a mixing bowl, combine the kale, scallions, avocado, sunflower seeds, lemon juice, olive oil, and salt, and pepper.

2. Combine well.

3. Mix the pomegranate seeds and serve fresh.

Nutritional Values (Per Serving):

Calories 243, Fat 18g, Carbohydrates 13g, Fiber 5g, Protein 6g

Black Bean Chili Potato

Recipe Time: 25 minutes

Serving Size: 7-8

Meal Type: Dinner

Diet Type: Gluten Free, Dairy Free, Soy Free, Nut Free, Vegan, Vegetarian

Ingredients:

- 1 red bell pepper, diced
- 1 green bell pepper, diced
- 3 cups cooked sweet potato cubes
- 2 tablespoons avocado oil
- 1 red onion, diced
- 5 garlic cloves, minced
- 1 (28-ounce) can diced tomatoes with their juice
- 1 tablespoon lime juice
- 3 cups cooked black beans, drained and rinsed well
- 2 cups vegetable broth
- 1 teaspoon ground cumin
- 1 teaspoon salt
- 1 tablespoon chili powder
- 1 teaspoon cocoa powder
- ½ teaspoon ground cinnamon

- ¼ teaspoon cayenne pepper

- ¼ teaspoon dried oregano

Cooking Instructions:

1. In a cooking pot (you can also use a deep saucepan); heat the oil over medium stove flame.

2. Add the onions, garlic, stir the mixture and cook while stirring for about 2-3 minutes until softened.

3. Add the red bell pepper and green bell pepper; stir-cook for about 3 minutes until soft.

4. Add the other ingredients and stir to combine.

5. Bring to a simmer, and cook for 15 minutes. Serve immediately.

Nutritional Values (Per Serving):

Calories 162, Fat 4g, Carbohydrates 28g, Fiber 6g, Protein 8g

Chickpea Veggie Lunch

Recipe Time: 35 minutes

Serving Size: 4

Meal Type: Lunch

Diet Type: Gluten Free, Dairy Free, Soy Free, Nut Free, Vegan, Vegetarian

Ingredients:

- 1 teaspoon sweet paprika

- 2 teaspoons turmeric powder

- 1 tablespoon coconut oil

- 15 ounces canned chickpeas, drained

- 8 small potatoes, cubed

- ¼ cup quinoa

- A pinch of (ground) black pepper and salt

- ½ tablespoon olive oil

- 2 kale leaves, chopped

- 1 avocado, pitted, peeled and sliced

Cooking Instructions:

1. Preheat an oven to 450°F. Line two baking sheets with a foil.

2. Place the potatoes on the sheet, drizzle the coconut oil over.

3. Sprinkle 1 teaspoon turmeric, and season with salt and pepper.

4. Bake for 5 minutes and set aside.

5. In a bowl (medium size), mix the chickpeas with the paprika, toss.

6. Place them over another baking sheet. Bake for 20 minutes at 350°F.

7. In a mixing bowl, mix the potatoes with the chickpeas.

8. Add the rest of the turmeric, olive oil, salt, pepper, quinoa, kale and avocado.

9. Toss and serve.

Nutritional Values (Per Serving):

Calories 291, Fat 4g, Carbohydrates 15g, Fiber 6g, Protein 8g

Fruit Blast Salad

Recipe Time: 15 minutes

Serving Size: 6

Meal Type: Lunch

Diet Type: Gluten Free, Dairy Free, Soy Free, Vegetarian

Ingredients:

- 1 cup nectarines, sliced
- ½ cup pecans, chopped
- ¼ cup red onion, thinly sliced
- 4 cups mixed chopped greens
- 1 cup peaches, sliced
- 1 cup cherries, pitted and halved
- ¼ cup basil leaves
- 1 tablespoon lemon juice
- ½ tablespoon raw honey
- ⅓ cup extra-virgin olive oil
- ¼ cup balsamic vinegar
- Dash salt and ground black pepper to taste

Cooking Instructions:

1. In a mixing bowl, combine the greens, peaches, cherries, nectarines, pecans, red onion, and basil.

2. In another bowl, add the olive oil, vinegar, lemon juice, honey, salt and pepper. Combine well.

3. Pour the dressing mix over the salad. Toss well and serve.

Nutritional Values (Per Serving):

Calories 219, Fat 18g, Carbohydrates 17g, Fiber 3g, Protein 2g

Avocado Quinoa Salad

Recipe Time: 5 minutes

Serving Size: 2

Meal Type: Lunch

Diet Type: Gluten Free, Dairy Free, Soy Free, Vegan, Vegetarian

Ingredients:

- 1 medium bunch collard greens, chopped
- 4 tablespoons walnuts, chopped
- 1 cup quinoa, cooked
- 1 avocado, chopped
- 2 tablespoons white wine vinegar
- 1 tablespoon olive oil
- 1 tablespoon maple syrup

Cooking Instructions:

1. In a bowl (medium size), combine the quinoa, avocado, greens, walnuts, vinegar, oil and maple syrup.

2. Toss well and serve.

Nutritional Values (Per Serving):

Calories 168, Fat 3g, Carbohydrates 6g, Fiber 2g, Protein 3g

Chickpea Patties

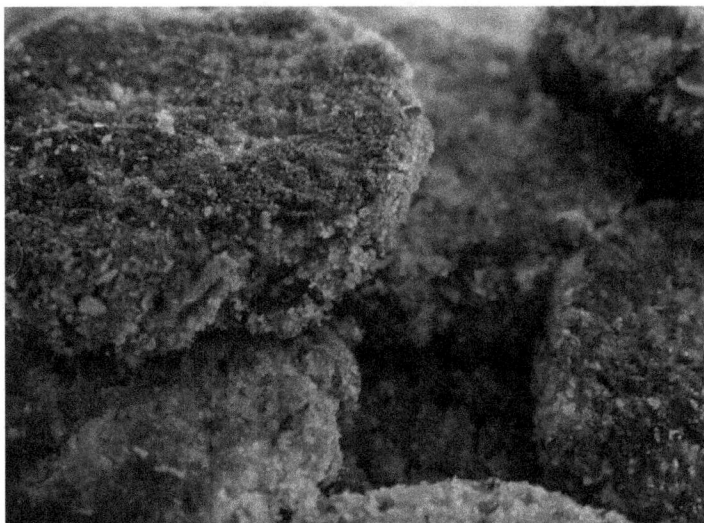

Recipe Time: 20 minutes

Serving Size: 4

Meal Type: Lunch

Diet Type: Gluten Free, Dairy Free, Soy Free, Nut Free, Vegan, Vegetarian

Ingredients:

- ¼ cup parsley leaves
- 2 tablespoons coconut flour
- 2 tablespoons chickpeas flour
- 2 garlic cloves, peeled
- 1 yellow onion, peeled and chopped

- 1 ½ cups canned chickpeas, drained and rinsed

- 1 teaspoon turmeric powder

- A pinch of (ground) black pepper and salt

- A pinch of cayenne pepper

- 3 tablespoons coconut or olive oil

Cooking Instructions:

1. In a blender, mix the garlic with the onion, chickpeas, parsley, coconut flour, turmeric, salt, pepper and cayenne.

2. Make patties from the mix. Coat them in the chickpeas flour.

3. In a skillet (you can also use a saucepan); heat the oil over medium stove flame.

4. Cook the patties for 4-5 minutes on each side.

5. Serve with your choice of dip or fresh chopped veggies.

Nutritional Values (Per Serving):

Calories 249, Fat 4g, Carbohydrates 14g, Fiber 4g, Protein 8g

Chickpea Raisin Curry

Recipe Time: 20 minutes

Serving Size: 4

Meal Type: Dinner

Diet Type: Gluten Free, Soy Free, Vegetarian

Ingredients:

- 1 red bell pepper, chopped

- 1 ½ cups vegetable broth

- 1 tablespoon curry powder

- 2 small white onions, diced

- 2 garlic cloves, minced

- 2 tablespoons avocado oil

- ½ teaspoon salt

- 2 cups cooked chickpeas, rinsed and drained

- ½ cup golden raisins

- 1 medium apple, diced

- ½ cup cashews, roughly chopped

- ½ cup plain whole-milk yogurt (optional)

Cooking Instructions:

1. In a skillet (you can also use a saucepan); heat the oil over medium stove flame.

2. Add the onions, garlic, stir the mixture and cook while stirring for about 2-3 minutes until softened.

3. Add the bell pepper, and sauté for 4-5 minutes.

4. Add the broth, curry powder, and salt; combine and bring to a simmer.

5. Add the chickpeas, apple, and raisins; cook for 4-5 minutes.

6. Mix in the cashews. Serve warm with the yogurt on top.

Nutritional Values (Per Serving):

Calories 378, Fat 17g, Carbohydrates 38g, Fiber 12g, Protein 11g

Zucchini Buckwheat Pasta

Recipe Time: 15 minutes

Serving Size: 4

Meal Type: Dinner

Diet Type: Gluten Free, Soy Free, Vegetarian

Ingredients:

Pesto:

- ¼ cup shelled sunflower seeds

- 2 garlic cloves

- 1 cup basil leaves

- 1 cup chopped zucchini

- ½ cup extra-virgin olive oil, divided

- ¼ cup raw Parmesan cheese, shredded

- 1 teaspoon lemon juice

- ¼ teaspoon salt

- Freshly ground black pepper

Pasta:

- 8 ounces buckwheat pasta

Cooking Instructions:

1. Cook the pasta in water as directed on pack.

2. In a food processor (or blender), puree the basil, zucchini, sunflower seeds, garlic, and ¼ cup of olive oil.

3. Add the cheese, lemon juice, salt, and pepper. Blend to combine well.

4. Add the remaining oil and blend well.

5. Serve the pesto with the pasta and top with sunflower seeds.

Nutritional Values (Per Serving):

Calories 426, Fat 25g, Carbohydrates 34g, Fiber 4g, Protein 9g

Brown Rice Lentils

Recipe Time: 30 minutes

Serving Size: 4

Meal Type: Dinner

Diet Type: Gluten Free, Dairy Free, Soy Free, Nut Free, Vegan, Vegetarian

Ingredients:

- 1 celery stalk, finely chopped
- 1 carrot, minced
- 2 garlic cloves, minced
- 2 tablespoons avocado oil
- 1 small white onion, chopped
- 7 tablespoons tomato paste
- 2 tablespoons apple cider vinegar
- 1 pound cooked lentils
- ½ red bell pepper, finely chopped
- 1 tablespoon pure maple syrup
- 1 teaspoon Dijon mustard
- 1 teaspoon chili powder
- ½ teaspoon dried oregano
- Cooked brown rice or wild rice to serve

Cooking Instructions:

1. In a skillet (you can also use a saucepan); heat the oil over medium stove flame.

2. Add the onion, celery, carrot, and garlic, stir the mixture and cook while stirring for about 4-5 minutes until softened.

3. Add the bell pepper, and sauté for 2 minutes.

4. Add the tomato paste, vinegar, maple syrup, mustard, chili powder, and oregano.

5. Reduce cooking flame and stir-cook for about 8-10 minutes.

6. Serve warm with the rice.

Nutritional Values (Per Serving):

Calories 288, Fat 7g, Carbohydrates 32g, Fiber 10g, Protein 14g

Mushroom Rice Bowl

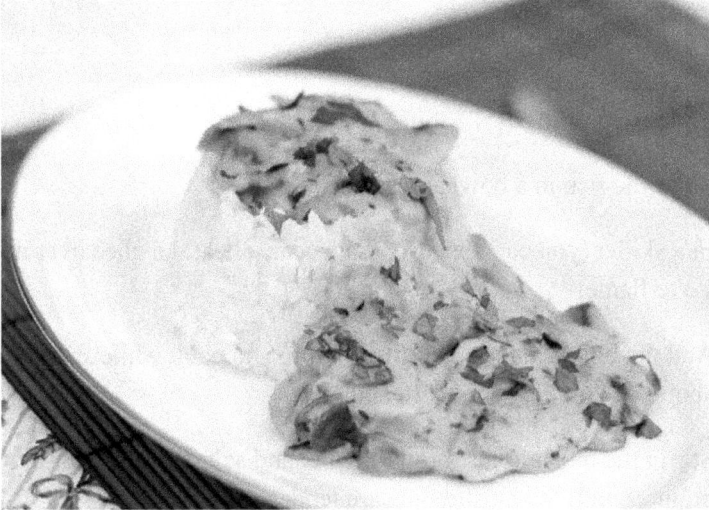

Recipe Time: 25 minutes

Serving Size: 8

Meal Type: Lunch

Diet Type: Gluten Free, Soy Free, Nut Free, Vegetarian

Ingredients:

- 1 small sweet onion, diced

- 3 garlic cloves, minced

- 2 cups cremini mushrooms, (cut into slices)

- 3 cups cooked wild rice

- 2 tablespoons ghee

- ½ cup vegetable broth

- ½ teaspoon dried thyme

- ½ teaspoon salt

Cooking Instructions:

1. Place the rice in a bowl and set aside.

2. In a skillet (you can also use a saucepan); heat the ghee over medium stove flame.

3. Add the onions, garlic, stir the mixture and cook while stirring for about 4-5 minutes until softened.

4. Stir in the mushrooms, broth, thyme, and salt; stir-cook for 8-10 minutes until the mushrooms are tender.

5. Add the mixture to the rice and serve warm.

Nutritional Values (Per Serving):

Calories 148, Fat 3g, Carbohydrates 23g, Fiber 2g, Protein 5g

Chickpea Lettuce Wraps

Recipe Time: 15 minutes

Serving Size: 2

Meal Type: Lunch or Dinner

Diet Type: Gluten Free, Dairy Free, Soy Free, Nut Free, Vegetarian

Ingredients:

- ½ shallot, minced
- 1 green apple, cored and diced
- 3 tablespoons tahini (sesame paste)
- 1 (15-ounce) can chickpeas, drained and rinsed well
- 1 celery stalk, diced
- 1 teaspoon Dijon mustard
- 2 teaspoons lemon juice
- 1 teaspoon raw honey
- Dash salt to taste
- 4 romaine lettuce leaves

Cooking Instructions:

1. In a bowl (medium size), combine the chickpeas, celery, shallot, apple, tahini, lemon juice, honey, mustard, and salt. Combine well.

2. Add the mix over the romaine lettuce leaves on a plate.

3. Wrap the leaves and serve.

Nutritional Values (Per Serving):

Calories 317, Fat 14g, Carbohydrates 31g, Fiber 12g, Protein 15g

Snacks & Sauces

Avocado Prosciutto Snack

Recipe Time: 5 minutes

Serving Size/Yield: 12

Diet Type: Gluten Free, Dairy Free, Soy Free, Nut Free

Ingredients:

- 2 large avocados, halved, pitted
- 12 slices prosciutto
- 2 apples, each cut into 6 pieces
- Raw honey (optional)

Cooking Instructions:

1. Take each avocado halves and make 3 slices from each half.

2. Take 1 prosciutto slice; place 1 avocado slice and 1 apple slice at one end and roll to make a wrap. Repeat the same.

3. Top with the honey and serve.

Nutritional Values (Per Serving):

Calories 238, Fat 17g, Carbohydrates 11g, Fiber 5g, Protein 16g

Honey Bean Dip

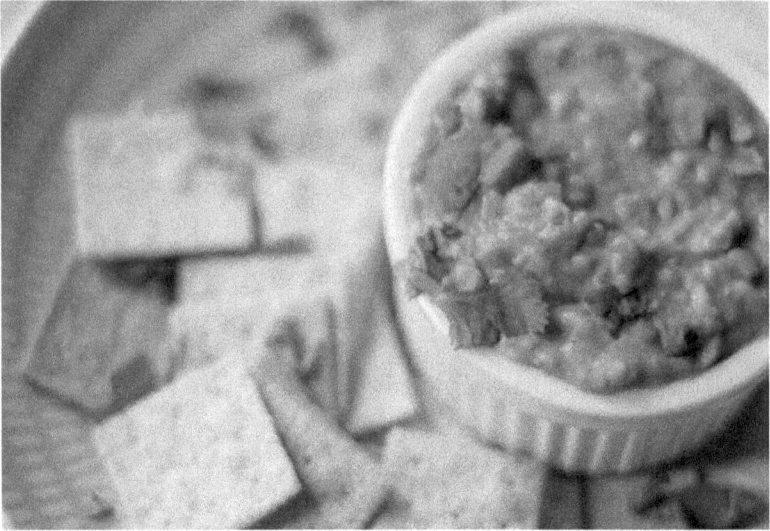

Recipe Time: 5 minutes

Serving Size/Yield: 3-4 cups

Diet Type: Gluten Free, Dairy Free, Soy Free, Nut Free, Vegetarian

Ingredients:

- 2 cherry tomatoes

- 2 tablespoons filtered water

- 1 tablespoon apple cider vinegar

- 1 (14-ounce) can each of kidney beans and black beans

- 2 garlic cloves

- ¼ teaspoon ground cumin

- ¼ teaspoon salt

- 2 teaspoons raw honey

- 1 teaspoon lime juice

- Pinch cayenne pepper to taste

- Freshly ground black pepper to taste

Cooking Instructions:

1. In a blender or food processor, add the beans, garlic, tomatoes, water, vinegar, honey, lime juice, cumin, salt, cayenne pepper, and black pepper.

2. Blend until turns smooth. Add the mix in a bowl.

3. Cover and refrigerate to chill. You can refrigerate for up to 5 days.

Nutritional Values (Per Serving ½ cup):

Calories 158, Fat 1g, Carbohydrates 33g, Fiber 8g, Protein 9g

Bean Potato Spread

Recipe Time: 25 minutes

Serving Size: 7-8

Diet Type: Gluten Free, Dairy Free, Soy Free, Nut Free, Vegan, Vegetarian

Ingredients:

- 2 tablespoons lime juice
- 1 tablespoon olive oil
- 5 garlic cloves, minced
- 1 cup canned garbanzo beans, drained and rinsed
- 4 cups cooked sweet potatoes, peeled and chopped
- ¼ cup sesame paste
- ½ teaspoon cumin, ground
- 2 tablespoons water
- A pinch of salt

Cooking Instructions:

1. In a blender, add all the ingredients and blend to make a smooth mix.

2. Transfer to a bowl.

3. Serve with carrot, celery or veggie sticks.

Nutritional Values (Per Serving):

Calories 156, Fat 3g, Carbohydrates 10g, Fiber 6g, Protein 8g

Zucchini Crisps

Recipe Time: 30 minutes

Serving Size/Yield: 12 pieces

Diet Type: Gluten Free, Soy Free, Nut Free, Vegan, Vegetarian

Ingredients:

- ½ cup almond flour
- 1 medium zucchini, peeled and halved widthwise
- 1 tablespoon avocado oil
- ½ teaspoon salt
- ½ teaspoon garlic powder
- ½ teaspoon ground black pepper

Cooking Instructions:

1. Preheat an oven to 425°F. Line a baking sheet with a foil.

2. In a mixing bowl, mix the flour, salt, garlic powder, and pepper.

3. Make total 12 strips from zucchini halves.

4. Brush the strips with the oil, and coat with the flour mixture. Evenly space the fries on the prepared sheet.

5. Bake for 20 minutes, or until crispy. Serve warm.

Nutritional Values (Per Piece):

Calories 42, Fat 3g, Carbohydrates 2g, Fiber 0.3g, Protein 1g

Evening Chicken Bites

Recipe Time: 20 minutes

Serving Size: 2

Diet Type: Gluten Free, Dairy Free, Soy Free

Ingredients:

- 2 tablespoons garlic powder

- 2 chicken breasts, cubed

- ½ cup almond flour

- 1 egg

- (ground) black pepper and salt to the taste

- ½ cup coconut oil

Cooking Instructions:

1. In a bowl (medium size), mix the garlic powder, flour, salt and pepper and stir.

2. In another bowl, whisk the egg.

3. Coat the chicken breast cubes in egg mix, then coat with the flour mix.

4. In a skillet (you can also use a saucepan); heat the oil over medium stove flame.

5. Add the chicken pieces, cook them for 4-5 minutes on each side until cooks well.

6. Serve warm.

Nutritional Values (Per Serving):

Calories 72, Fat 4g, Carbohydrates 6g, Fiber 2g, Protein 8g

Cashew Ginger Dip

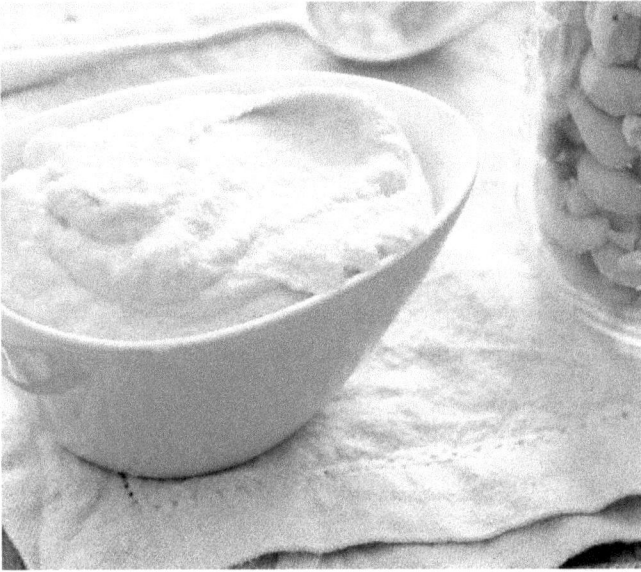

Recipe Time: 5 minutes

Serving Size/Yield: 1 cup

Diet Type: Gluten Free, Dairy Free, Soy Free, Vegan, Vegetarian

Ingredients:

- 1 tablespoon extra-virgin olive oil

- 2 teaspoons coconut aminos

- 1 cup raw cashews, soaked in filtered water for 20-25 minutes and drained

- 2 garlic cloves

- ¼ cup filtered water

- 1 teaspoon lemon juice

- ½ teaspoon ground ginger

- ¼ teaspoon salt

- Pinch cayenne pepper

Cooking Instructions:

1. In a blender or food processor, puree the cashews, garlic, water, olive oil, aminos, lemon juice, ginger, salt, and cayenne pepper.

2. Add the mix in a bowl.

3. Cover and refrigerate until chilled. You can use store it for 4-5 days in refrigerator.

Nutritional Values (Per Serving):

Calories 124, Fat 9g, Carbohydrates 5g, Fiber 1g, Protein 3g

Buckwheat Evening Delight

Recipe Time: 25 minutes

Serving Size: 4

Diet Type: Gluten Free, Dairy Free, Soy Free, Nut Free, Vegan, Vegetarian

Ingredients:

- 2 teaspoons minced garlic

- 2 cups cooked buckwheat

- 1 tablespoon olive oil

- ½ cup chopped red onion

- Juice of 1 lemon

- Zest of 1 lemon (optional)

- ½ cup chopped parsley

- ¼ cup chopped mint

- Sea salt to taste

Cooking Instructions:

1. In a skillet (you can also use a saucepan); heat the oil over medium stove flame.

2. Add the onions, garlic, stir the mixture and cook while stirring for about 2-3 minutes until softened.

3. Stir in the buckwheat, lemon juice, and lemon zest. Stir-cook for about 4-5 minutes.

4. Stir in the parsley and mint. Sauté for 1 minute.

5. Remove from the heat and season with salt. Serve warm.

Nutritional Values (Per Serving):

Calories 394, Fat 6g, Carbohydrates 38g, Fiber 9g, Protein 16g

Spiced Chickpeas

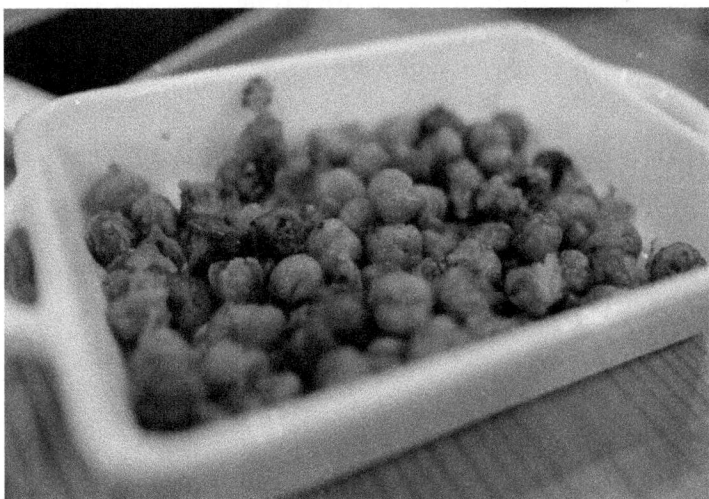

Recipe Time: 20-25 minutes

Serving Size/Yield: 4 cups

Diet Type: Gluten Free, Dairy Free, Soy Free, Nut Free, Vegan, Vegetarian

Ingredients:

- 4 cups cooked chickpeas, drained, and dried

- 1 teaspoon garlic powder

- 2 tablespoons extra-virgin olive oil

- 1 teaspoon salt

- Ground black pepper to taste

Cooking Instructions:

1. Preheat an oven to 400°F. Line a baking sheet with a foil.

2. Spread the chickpeas and coat with the oil.

3. Bake for 20 minutes, shake it in between.

4. Add them to a large bowl.

5. Toss with the salt and garlic powder; season with pepper. Serve warm.

Nutritional Values (Per Serving ¼ cup):

Calories 148, Fat 5g, Carbohydrates 22g, Fiber 6g, Protein 8g

Desserts

Blackberry Granita

Recipe Time: 10 minutes

Serving Size: 4

Diet Type: Gluten Free, Dairy Free, Soy Free, Nut Free, Vegetarian

Ingredients:

- ½ cup raw honey
- ¼ cup lemon juice
- 1 pound blackberries
- ½ cup water
- 1 teaspoon chopped thyme

Cooking Instructions:

1. In a blender or food processor, combine the blackberries, water, honey, lemon juice, and thyme.

2. Blend to make a smooth puree.

3. Process through a fine-mesh sieve into a square baking dish. D

4. Place it in the freezer for 2 hours. Remove the dish and break any frozen section by stirring gently. Free again for 1-2 hours; repeat the same until you get a granite like structure.

5. Serve chilled.

Nutritional Values (Per Serving):

Calories 176, Fat 1g, Carbohydrates 42g, Fiber 6g, Protein 2g

Spiced Fruit Blast

Recipe Time: 35 minutes

Serving Size: 4

Diet Type: Gluten Free, Dairy Free, Soy Free, Vegan, Vegetarian

Ingredients:

For Filling:

- 1 large mango, peeled and diced

- 1 pineapple, peeled and cut into small chunks

- 2 tablespoons coconut oil

- 2 tablespoons maple syrup

- 1/8 teaspoon ground cinnamon

- 1/8 teaspoon ground ginger

For Topping:

- ½ teaspoon ground allspice

- ½ teaspoon ground cinnamon

- ½ teaspoon ground ginger

- ¾ cup almonds

- 1/3 cup coconut, shredded

Cooking Instructions:

1. Preheat an oven to 375°F. Grease a baking dish with some cooking spray.

2. In a skillet (you can also use a saucepan); heat the oil over medium stove flame.

3. Add the maple syrup and cook, stirring for about 1-2 minutes.

4. Stir in remaining ingredients and cook for 4-5 minutes.

5. Remove from heat, cool down and add into a baking dish.

6. In a blender, add the topping ingredients.

7. Blend to make a meal like mixture.

8. Bake for about 15 minutes or turns golden brown. Serve warm.

Nutritional Values (Per Serving):

Calories 307, Fat 22g, Carbohydrates 26g, Fiber 4g, Protein 3g

Cherry Cobbler

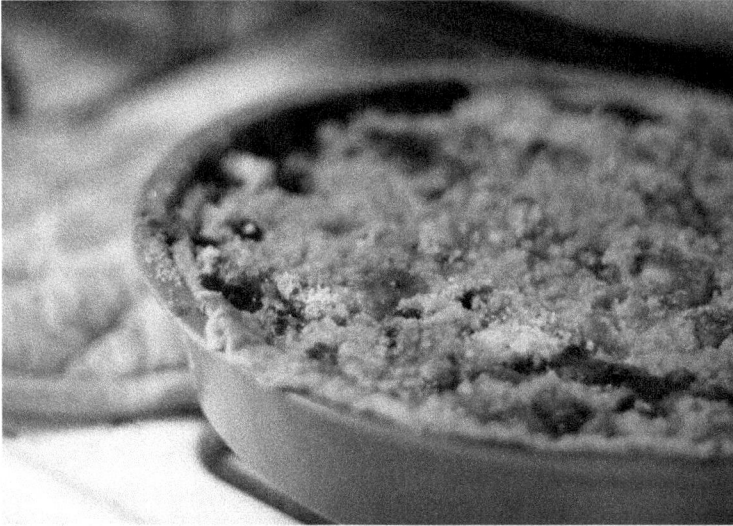

Recipe Time: 30-35 minutes

Serving Size: 4

Diet Type: Gluten Free, Dairy Free, Soy Free, Nut Free, Vegan, Vegetarian

Ingredients:

- ¼ cup unsweetened coconut, shredded

- ¼ cup coconut flour

- 1 tablespoon arrowroot flour

- 2 cups cherries, pitted

- ¼ cup +1 tablespoon cup maple syrup

- ¼ cup pecans, chopped

- ½ teaspoon ground cinnamon

- Pinch of salt

Cooking Instructions:

1. Preheat an oven to 375°F. Grease a baking dish with some cooking spray.

2. Add the cherries and ¼ cup syrup.

3. In a bowl (medium size), combine the 1 tablespoon of maple syrup and remaining ingredients.

4. Add the mixture over cherries evenly.

5. Bake for 25 minutes and serve warm.

Nutritional Values (Per Serving):

Calories 168, Fat 13g, Carbohydrates 22g, Fiber 1g, Protein 5g

Lemon Coconut Mousse

Recipe Time: 15-20 minutes

Serving Size: 4

Diet Type: Gluten Free, Dairy Free, Soy Free, Nut Free, Vegetarian

Ingredients:

- 2 cups coconut milk

- ½ cup lemon juice

- ¼ cup water

- 2 teaspoons powdered gelatin

- ¼ cup raw honey

- 2 tablespoons lemon zest

Cooking Instructions:

1. In a skillet (you can also use a saucepan); heat the water over medium stove flame.

2. Mix in the gelatin and set aside for 10 minutes to thicken.

3. In a bowl (medium size), whisk the milk, lemon juice, honey, and lemon zest.

4. Heat the gelatin mix again and add the milk mixture; stir and heat the mixture.

5. Cool down and refrigerate for about 2 hours until set.

6. Add the mousse into serving bowls.

Nutritional Values (Per Serving):

Calories 318, Fat 11g, Carbohydrates 26g, Fiber 4g, Protein 3g

Quinoa Dessert Bars

Recipe Time: 10 minutes

Serving Size: 8

Diet Type: Gluten Free, Dairy Free, Soy Free, Vegetarian

Ingredients:

- ¼ cup raw honey

- ¼ cup cocoa powder

- ½ cup almond butter

- 4 cups puffed quinoa

- ¼ cup chopped almonds

Cooking Instructions:

1. Grease a square baking dish with some cooking spray.

2. In a skillet (you can also use a saucepan); heat the butter over medium stove flame.

3. Add the honey and cocoa powder. Stir and heat the mix; set aside to cool down.

4. In a mixing bowl, toss the quinoa and almonds.

5. Add the pan mixture. Stir everything together.

6. Add the mixture into the dish and press firmly.

7. Refrigerate for about 1-2 hour. Slice into 16 pieces and serve.

Nutritional Values (Per Serving):

Calories 96, Fat 3g, Carbohydrates 17g, Fiber 1g, Protein 2g

Apple Pear Delight

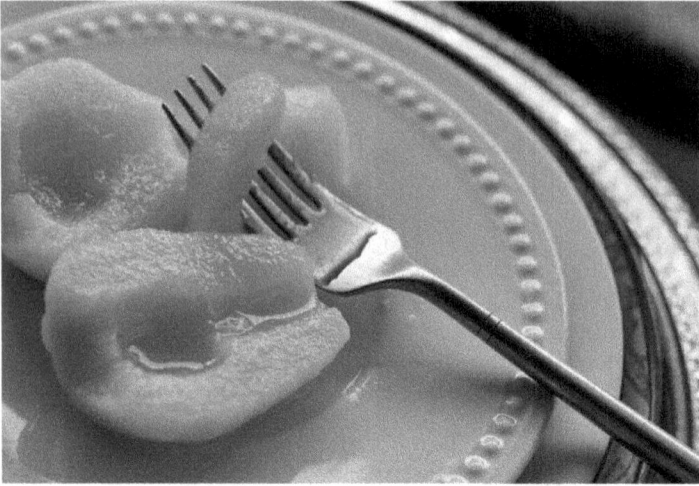

Recipe Time: 25 minutes

Serving Size: 4

Diet Type: Gluten Free, Dairy Free, Soy Free, Nut Free, Vegetarian

Ingredients:

- ¼ cup raw honey

- 1 teaspoon whole cloves

- 4 cups water

- 2 cups unsweetened apple juice

- ½ teaspoon whole cardamom seeds

- 1 teaspoon pure vanilla extract

- 4 pears, peeled, cored and halved

Cooking Instructions:

1. In a skillet (you can also use a saucepan); heat the honey, cloves, water, apple juice, cardamom, and vanilla over medium stove flame.

2. Boil the mix. Reduce the heat to low and simmer for 5 minutes.

3. Add the pear and cover. Simmer for about 8-10 minutes, stirring in between.

4. Add the mixture in serving plates. Serve the pears with the liquid sauce on top.

Nutritional Values (Per Serving):

Calories 238, Fat 0g, Carbohydrates 52g, Fiber 7g, Protein 1g

Pumpkin Pecan Treat

Recipe Time: 10 minutes

Serving Size: 6

Diet Type: Gluten Free, Dairy Free, Soy Free, Nut Free, Vegan, Vegetarian

Ingredients:

1 teaspoon ground cinnamon

½ teaspoon ground ginger

¼ teaspoon ground nutmeg

2 cups canned full-fat coconut milk

1 cup pure pumpkin purée

¼ cup pure maple syrup

Pinch cloves

2 tablespoons chopped pecans, for garnish

Cooking Instructions:

1. In a mixing bowl, whisk the milk, cinnamon, ginger, pumpkin, maple syrup, nutmeg, and cloves.

2. Cover it and refrigerator the bowl for about 2 hours until chilled.

3. Top with the pecans and serve.

Nutritional Values (Per Serving):

Calories 246, Fat 18g, Carbohydrates 17g, Fiber 3g, Protein 4g

Conclusion

Thanks again for taking your valuable time to read this book!

Inflammation fighting foods inspire impactful life changes. They bring true nutrition to your dining table every day. Environmental stimuli affect our gene structure and triggers our body's natural defense through auto-immune response.

Inflammation is the root cause of number of health disorders and ailments. Thankfully, we have the power fight against them by following a wholesome diet. These health diet changes help to relieved the symptoms of auto-immune diseases including arthritis and join pain.

The recipes covered in the book are satiating and full of vibrant flavors. Meal plan is really helpful for beginners as they can consume meals combining various vegetables, spices, meats, and fish varieties.

As you know all the anti-inflammatory foods that you can include in your diet; you can experiment with every day recipes. You can add your choice of ingredients to customize flavors of your preference.

What are you waiting for? Make a trip to your nearby supermarket, stuff your pantry with anti-inflammatory ingredients, and start making these delicious recipes. Thank you and have a great time enjoying these wholesome recipes!

Lastly, if you enjoyed this book, please take the time to review it on Amazon. Your honest feedback would be greatly appreciated. Wish you all the best in achieving vibrancy and optimal health that you all deserve.

Have a great day! Best of luck in all your endeavors.

The Anti-Inflammatory Slow Cooker Recipes

Step by Step Guide With 130+ Proven Slow Cooking Recipes for Immune System Healing and Overall Health

John Carter

Text Copyright © John Carter

Legal & Disclaimer

The information contained in this book and its contents is not designed to replace or take the place of any form of medical or professional advice; and is not meant to replace the need for independent medical, financial, legal or other professional advice or services, as may be required. The content and information in this book has been provided for educational and entertainment purposes only.

The content and information contained in this book has been compiled from sources deemed reliable, and it is accurate to the best of the Author's knowledge, information and belief. However, the Author cannot guarantee its accuracy and validity and cannot be held liable for any errors and/or omissions. Further, changes are periodically made to this book as and when needed. Where appropriate and/or necessary, you must consult a professional (including but not limited to your doctor, attorney, financial advisor or such other professional advisor) before using any of the suggested remedies, techniques, or information in this book.

Upon using the contents and information contained in this book, you agree to hold harmless the Author from and against any damages, costs, and expenses, including any legal fees potentially resulting from the application of any of the information provided by this book. This disclaimer applies to any loss, damages or injury caused by the use and application, whether directly or indirectly, of any advice or information presented, whether for breach of contract, tort, negligence, personal injury, criminal intent, or under any other cause of action.

You agree to accept all risks of using the information presented inside this book.

You agree that by continuing to read this book, where appropriate and/or necessary, you shall consult a professional (including but not limited to your doctor, attorney, or financial advisor or such other advisor as needed) before using any of the suggested remedies, techniques, or information in this book.

Table of Contents

Introduction:
Understanding Inflammation and Anti-Inflammatory Diet Recipes

Why Do We Need Anti-Inflammatory Diet

What is Inflammation and What It Does to Your Body?

Inflammation is a process by which white blood cells along with the substances they produce protects the body from invading external organisms like viruses and bacteria. However, there are instances when the body defense system - which is the immune system - triggers an inflammatory response even in the absence of a foreign invasion. Without the enemy to fight off, the immune system causes harm to its own tissues, hence the onset of autoimmune diseases like arthritis. But not all arthritis is caused by misguided inflammation. Arthritis that is usually associated with inflammation is:

- Psoriatic arthritis

- Rheumatoid arthritis

- Gouty arthritis

Symptoms of Inflammation include:

- Swollen joints and pain

- Loss of joint function and stiffness

- Redness in the external area surrounding the affected joints

Inflammation is also a form of defense mechanism. As the body's immune system recognizes damage cells, pathogens, and irritant, it resorts to healing itself. It is part of the body's immune response and without inflammation; any damage to tissues would not be able to heal without it.

However, once it becomes chronic, it can become harmful to the human body. Chronic inflammation is recurring and can last for years, leading to various damaging illnesses. Chronic inflammation can also occur in the body without the host being aware of it. This time of inflammation can drive death-leading conditions including

- Diabetes

- Cardiovascular disease

- Fatty liver disease

People suffering from stress and obesity are more prone to chronic inflammation.

Benefits of Embracing the Anti-Inflammatory Diet

An anti-inflammatory diet contains different nutrient-dense foods packed with antioxidants aims to reduce inflammatory responses. Antioxidants are reactive molecules in foods that combat free radicals. With these a large number of free radicals inside the body, it can damage cells and therefore increase the risk of certain diseases.

The Role of Inflammatory Diet

If you want to get away from chronic inflammation, there are foods that you need to eat and those that you need to avoid. It is essential that you need to base your diet on foods that filled with nutrients and contain antioxidants. Completely avoid processed food and eat foods that are closest to their natural state or those that are minimally processed.

Anti-Inflammatory Diet is used as a complementary therapy for many medical conditions worsened by chronic inflammation. Among them are:

- Asthma

- Psoriasis

- Rheumatoid arthritis

- Colitis

- Crohn's disease

- Eosinophilic esophagitis

- Lupus

- Metabolic syndrome

- Diabetes

- Obesity

- Inflammatory bowel disease

- Heart disease

- Hashimoto disease

- Certain cancers including colorectal cancer

What Foods to Eat and Foods to Avoid?

There are certain foods that should be part of your diet as they help reduce inflammatory risks.

- Tomatoes
- Olive Oil
- Nuts
- Leafy green vegetables like kale and spinach
- Fatty fish
- Fruits especially berries and oranges

Foods to Avoid

There are foods that can trigger chronic inflammation risk. Here are some of them

Refined Carbohydrates

- White bread
- White Pasta

Sugary Beverages and Alcoholic Drinks

- Soda
- Energy drinks
- Fruit juices
- Wine and liquors in an excessive amount

Processed Foods

- Desserts
- Cakes
- Candies
- Cookies
- Ice Cream
- Processed meats (hot dogs, sausages, ham, bolognas, etc.)

Processed Snack Foods

- Crackers
- Chips
- Other junk foods

Trans Fat and Certain Oils

- Processed oils from seeds and vegetables (corn oil, vegetable oils, etc.)
- Trans fats (Foods containing partially hydrogenated ingredients)

Important Tips to Follow

For some people, adjusting to an anti-inflammatory diet can be a big challenge. There are several things you can do to make this transition to an inflammatory diet easier.

- Eat more fruits and vegetables in a variety
- Keep away from eating fast foods
- Eliminate drinking soda and sugary drinks
- Plan your shopping list in advance to ensure that you will be buying healthful food and snacks
- Drink more water or lemon water
- Exercise regularly
- Male small anti-inflammatory snacks on hand and ready any time
- Have a regular exercise regimen
- Maintain the daily calorie requirements
- Add supplements like omega-3 fat and turmeric to the diet

Introducing Slow Cooking and its Benefits

While the slow cooker may not have a diverse cooking task, yet it has many significant benefits, which are the primary reason why we write this book. So, before diving into cooking preparation of the Inflammatory Diet, learn the different benefits of using a slow cooker.

- Slow cooking in low temperature retains the necessary nutrients that are most volatile and lessen the chance of scorching foods as bits tend to stick to the bottom of the pan when cooking in an oven.

- The extended cooking hours allows better distribution of flavors in foods you are cooking

- Less expensive meats including roast, chuck steaks, and less-lean stewing beef can get tenderer with the long process of cooking. It is also a great way of cooking venison dishes.

- It allows you to free your oven and stove tops for other uses.

- It saves you energy and therefore lessens your budget compared to using a standard electric oven.

- It's convenient to use as you can just plug it and leave it unattended for all day.

The best things in life take time and patience, especially in food preparation. Those that are tastiest like stews are proof that while it takes a while to make, it may be one of the simplest to put together whether or not you have the time to spare.

Some Tricks and Safety Tips to Make Slow Cooking a Success

Here are few tips and tricks to help you brew or stew using your slow cooker.

You Can Cook Even Without a Recipe

Slow cooking or braising is a great way to improvise and as long as you put the stew's basic ingredients in the slow cooker, you will always manage to get things right. As a guide, understand that protein plus aromatics plus liquid equals stew.

Try combining flavors that blend together like beef chunk with red wine, short ribs, rosemary, thyme, ginger, sesame oil, pork shoulder, sweet soy sauce, grainy mustard, beer, and pepper.

Slow cookers when used correctly as perfectly safe to use. Since different foods have different cooking requirements, you can find many different slow cookers in the market. Nonetheless, it is important to follow the manufacturer's guide and instruction when using it.

Poultry and Frozen Meat Must Be Thawed First

Completely thaw frozen and poultry meat before placing it inside the slow cooker. Remember to thaw meat in the refrigerator so it can thaw but not warm enough for bacteria to feast on it and breed quickly. This way the meat is safe and gives it a better texture.

Tougher and less expensive pieces of meat like a lamb's shoulder are better cooked in slow cooker. Aside from it being great for cooking stews, casseroles, and other dishes, it allows enough time for the meaty favor to develop in a dish.

You Don't Need to Check every time When Cooking

Slow cookers can thoroughly cook when set correctly even without you doing close monitoring on your dish. There is no need to open the pot once it's turned on. Also, avoid removing the lid cover to avoid releasing steam bringing the temperature down which can affect the cooking time. A lot of steam can build up in the slow cooker so you have to be careful when removing the cover as it can give you a nasty burn.

What Foods Must Not be Cooked in a Slow Cooker?

There are certain beans including cannellini beans and raw red kidney beans contain phytohemagglutinin, a chemical substance that is destroyed through boiling. If not, it will cause you to get poisoned. Slow cooking won't have this effect on beans because of its regulated temperature. Completely cook the kidney beans first if you intend to include them in the dish.

You Can Reheat Food Only Once

When you need to reheat food cooked in a slow cooker, you can do it only once. It is always dangerous to reheat them after this.

Amazingly Delicious Recipes to Beat Inflammation

Breakfast

Anti-Inflammatory Breakfast Quinoa

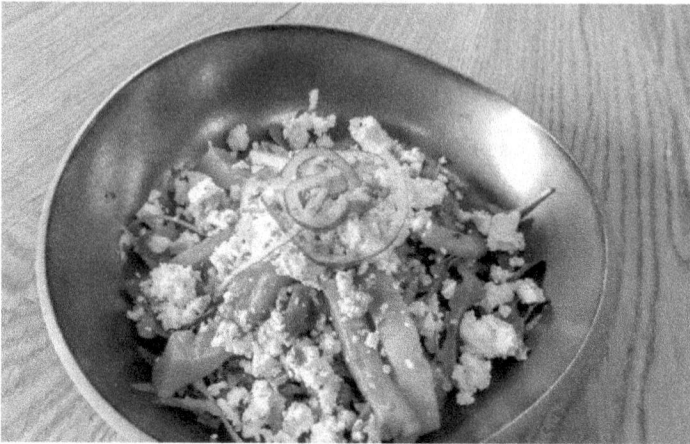

Ingredients

- 1 cup Quinoa
- 1 Apple, peeled and diced
- ¼ cup Pepitas
- 4 Medjool dates, chopped
- 3 cups Almond milk
- 2 tsp. Cinnamon
- 1 tsp. Vanilla extract
- ¼ tsp. Nutmeg
- ¼ tsp. Salt

Directions

1. Put all the ingredients into the crockpot and put the lid. Set on high and cook for 2 hours or until all the liquid has evaporated. (**Note:** If you want to cook it overnight, set it on low before going to bed.

Serving: 5

Nutritional Facts: Calories - 287; Carbohydrates - 50g; Fat - 5g; Protein - 12g

Banana & Coconut Milk Steel-Cut Oatmeal

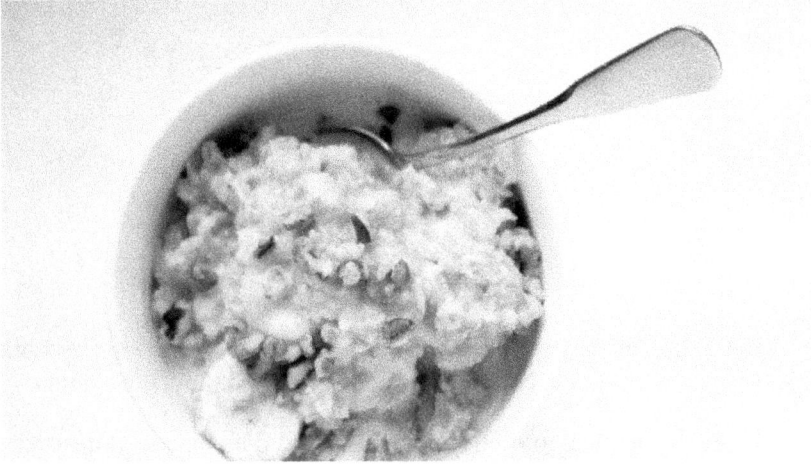

Ingredients

- 2 cups (about 2 medium-sized) Ripe bananas, sliced

- 1 cup Steel-cut oats

- 2 x 14-oz. cans of Light coconut milk

- ½ cup Water

- 1 ½ tbsp. Butter, cut into 5-6 pieces

- 1 tbsp. Ground flax seed

- ½ tsp. Cinnamon

- ½ tsp. Vanilla

- ¼ tsp. Nutmeg

- ¼ tsp. Salt

For garnish (optional):

- Bananas, sliced

- Walnuts, chopped

- Coconut, toasted

Directions

1. Lightly grease the crock with nonstick cooking spray.

2. Put all the ingredients (except for the toppings) to the slow cooker. Mix well, cover the cooker with lid, and cook on low for 7 hours.

3. Ladle the oatmeal into serving bowls. Add the toppings if desired.

Serving: 7 (serving size of ¾ cup)

Nutritional Facts: Calories - 373; Carbohydrates - 30.34g; Fats - 30.2g; Protein - 5.97g

Cardamom Orange Quinoa Bowl

Ingredients

- 1 cup Quinoa rice, cleansed
- 1 lb. Carrots, peeled and sliced
- 2 Oranges
- 1 tsp. Ground cardamom
- 2 ½ cups Chicken (or vegetable/ bone) broth
- ⅓ cup Golden raisins
- 1 x 1-inch pc. Fresh ginger, peeled and minced
- ½ tsp. Salt
- ½ tsp. Freshly ground black pepper

Directions

1. First, zest the oranges and set aside the fruit.

2. Put the quinoa, carrots, raisins, orange zest, ginger, cardamom, salt, black pepper, and broth in the slow cooker. Mix to combine. Cover the cooker with its lid and cook on low setting for about 3 to 3 ½ hours or until the quinoa is tender.

3. When the quinoa mix is nearly cooked, get the oranges. Peel off what remained in orange skins using a knife.

4. Once done with peeling off the skin, divide the orange into segments. To do this, work over a large bowl. Hold the orange on your non-dominant hand and hold a paring knife on your dominant hand. Slice between the membranes and let them drop into the bowl below. Continue until you're done with the oranges.

5. Scoop quinoa into serving bowls and garnish with oranges. Serve while hot.

Serving: 4

Nutritional Facts: Calories - 170; Carbohydrates - 31g; Fats - 3g; Protein - 5g

Creamy Slow-Cooked Yogurt

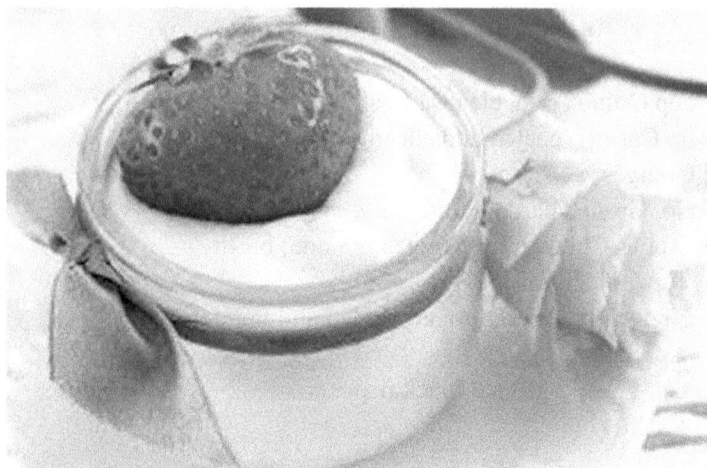

Ingredients

- ½ gallon Organic milk

- 3 tsp. Grass-fed gelatin

- 6 oz. Plain, organic yogurt with live cultures

Directions

1. Pour the milk into the slow cooker and cook on low for 3 hours or until the temperature reaches 150-175°F.

2. Ladle about 1 cup of milk into a bowl and add gelatin, 1 tsp. at a time. Whisk constantly to avoid any lumps. Return the mixture into the cooker and continue to whisk. (Note: In case of lumps, pour the mixture over a fine mesh strainer as you transfer it to the cooker.)

3. Turn the cooker off and allow the milk to rest for about 3 hours or until the mixture cools to about 110°F. (Note: If you put the yogurt starter when the temperature is still 115° or above, the bacteria will be damaged.)

4. Ladle 1 cup of milk from the cooker to a bowl and stir in the yogurt starter. Return the mixture to the cooker and gently mix.

5. Cover the entire cooker with a large blanket or a couple of large towels for about 10-12 hours. This will incubate the starters. (Note: If your kitchen is cooler than 70°, put a heat lamp near the cooker.)

6. Set aside 6 oz. of yogurt if you would make another batch of yogurt, this will be your starter. Refrigerate the rest to firm up. Enjoy!

Serving: 8

Nutritional Facts: Calories - 157; Carbohydrates - 11.83g; Fats - 8.11g; Protein - 9.38g

Greek Eggs Breakfast Casserole

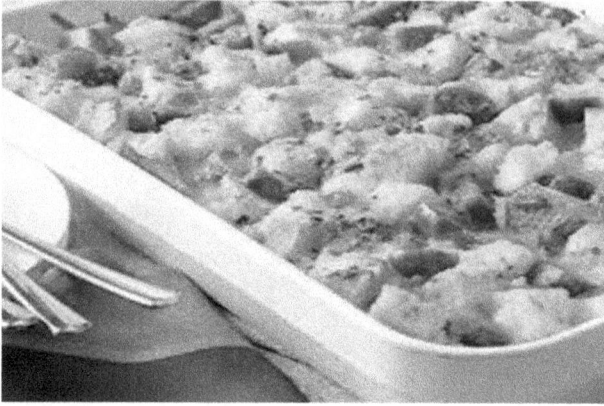

Ingredients

- 2 cups Spinach
- 1 cup Baby Bella mushrooms, sliced
- ½ cup Sun-dried tomatoes
- ½ cup Feta Cheese
- ½ cup Milk
- 1 tbsp. Red Onion
- 1 tsp. Garlic
- ½ tsp. Salt
- 1 tsp. Black pepper

Directions

1. In a large mixing bowl, whisk the eggs, salt, and pepper together. Add the mushrooms, tomatoes, spinach, onions, and garlic.

2. Stir the egg mixture and pour into the crock. Add the feta cheese on top and cook on low for about 4-6 hrs.

Serving: 4

Nutritional Facts: Calories - 81; Carbohydrates - 5.6g; Fats - 4.6g; Protein - 5g

Healthy Breakfast Casserole

Ingredients

- 1 Small broccoli head, roughly chopped
- 1 x 30-oz. bag Frozen hash browns
- 6 oz. Cheddar cheese (organic)
- 8 Whole eggs
- 4 Egg whites
- ¾ cup Milk
- 2 Bell peppers, roughly chopped
- ½ Onion, roughly chopped
- 2 tsp. Stone ground mustard
- ½ tsp. Garlic salt
- 1 tsp. Salt
- ½ tsp. Pepper

Directions

1. Whisked the milk, white eggs, whole eggs, garlic salt, mustard, salt, and pepper in a medium-sized mixing bowl then set aside.

2. Lightly coat the bottom of the crock with nonstick spray.

3. Arrange half of the hash browns at the bottom of the crock. Layer with half of the broccoli, bell peppers, onions, and cheese. Place the remaining of the hash browns and top with the rest of the veggies and cheese. Once done, pour the egg mixture on top.

4. Cover with lid and cook on low for about 4 hours. Serve hot.

Serving: 8

Nutritional Facts (per slice): Calories - 320; Carbohydrates - 29g; Fats - 13g; Protein - 22.1g

Pork Teriyaki Breakfast Rice Bowl

Ingredients

- 1 lb. Pork tenderloin, thinly sliced
- 2 cups Brown rice, washed
- 1 cups Mixed vegetables
- 3 cups Stock
- ½ cups Soy sauce
- tbsp. Ginger, grated
- ½ cups Honey
- tbsp. Grass-fed butter
- 1 tsp. Garlic, grated
- ¼ cups Mirin
- ½ cups Leeks, chopped

Directions

1. Mix the honey, soy sauce, mirin, garlic, and ginger in a bowl. Add the pork and marinate for 1 hour.

2. After an hour, put the pork (with marinade), rice, and stock into the cooker. Set to high and cook for about 2 hours.

3. Add the vegetables and leeks in the last 10 minutes of cooking time.

Serving: 8

Nutritional Facts: Calories - 400; Carbohydrates - 58.6g; Fats - 8.37g; Protein - 23g

Raspberry Chocolate Chip French Toast Casserole

Ingredients

- 5-6 cups Whole grain challah, cubed
- 1 cup Milk
- ½ cup Dark chocolate chips
- large Eggs
- ½ pint Raspberries
- 2 tbsp. Honey
- 1 tsp. Vanilla

Directions

1. In a medium bowl, stir in the eggs, honey, milk, and vanilla.

2. Put the challah cubes into a slow cooker and slightly push them down the cooker. Add the chocolate chips and half of the raspberries. Repeat to make another layer.

3. Pour the milk mixture on top. Cover the cooker with lid, set to high, and cook for about 2 hours or until the casserole has puffed up and turned golden.

Serving: 5

Nutritional Facts: Calories - 314; Carbohydrates - 33.8g; Fats - 15.5g; Protein - 9.7g

Simple Slow-Cooker Oatmeal

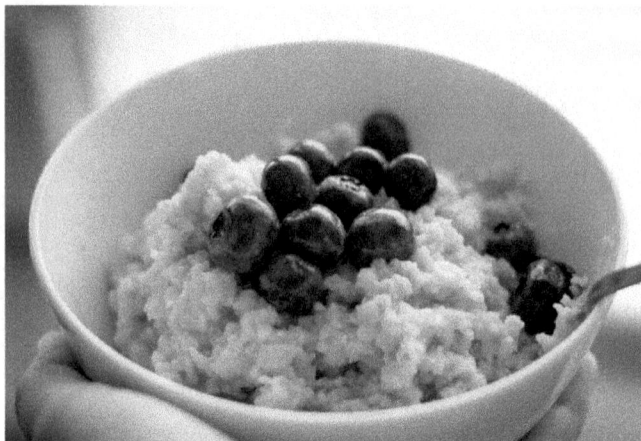

Ingredients

- 1 cup Steel-cut oats
- 4 cups Water
- ½ cup Grassmilk half and half
- 1 cup Dried cranberries (or blueberries)
- 1 cup Dates, chopped
- 2 tbsp. Honey

Directions

1. Lightly grease the crock of the slow cooker with nonstick spray.

2. Place oats, water, cranberries (or blueberries), and dates into the cooker. Secure cover and cook on low for about 7-8 hours.

3. Once done, stir in the honey and half & half. Serve and enjoy.

Serving: 4

Nutritional Facts: Calories - 157; Carbohydrates - 33g; Fats - 3g; Protein - 2g

Slow Cooker Apple Granola Crumble

Ingredients

- 2 Granny Smith apples, peeled, cored, and chunked
- 1 cup Granola
- ¼ cup Apple juice
- ⅛ cup Maple syrup
- 2 tbsp. Dairy-free butter
- ½ tsp. Ground nutmeg
- 1 tsp. Ground cinnamon

Directions

1. Add all the ingredients into the crock and mix well. Cover with lid and cook on low for about 4 hours.

Serving: 3

Nutritional Facts: Calories - 369; Carbohydrates - 56g; Fats - 15g; Protein - 5g

Slow-Cooked Apple Pie Amaranth Porridge

Ingredients

- 2 cups Amaranth, sprouted or soaked
- 5 Sweet apples, cored, diced
- 15 Large dates pitted
- 4 tbsp. Orange juice
- 1 cup Coconut milk
- 2 ½ cups Water
- 1 tbsp. Ground cinnamon
- ½ tsp. Ground nutmeg
- 1 tbsp. Vanilla extract

For the toppings (optional):

- Honey
- Nuts, chopped
- Raisins
- Goji berries

Directions

1 Coat the crock of the slow cooker with butter or coconut oil.

2 Put the ingredients into the slow cooker in this order: apples, date, cinnamon, nutmeg, vanilla extract, orange juice, amaranth, coconut milk, and water.

3   Cook overnight (to be served on breakfast the next day) or for about 8 hours on low setting.

4   Serve with your preferred toppings if desired.

5   Serving: 8 (serving size of ½ cup)

Nutritional Facts (per ½ cup, without the toppings): Calories - 343; Carbohydrates - 60g; Fats - 9.7g; Protein - 7.8g

Slow-Cooked Spinach and Mozzarella Frittata

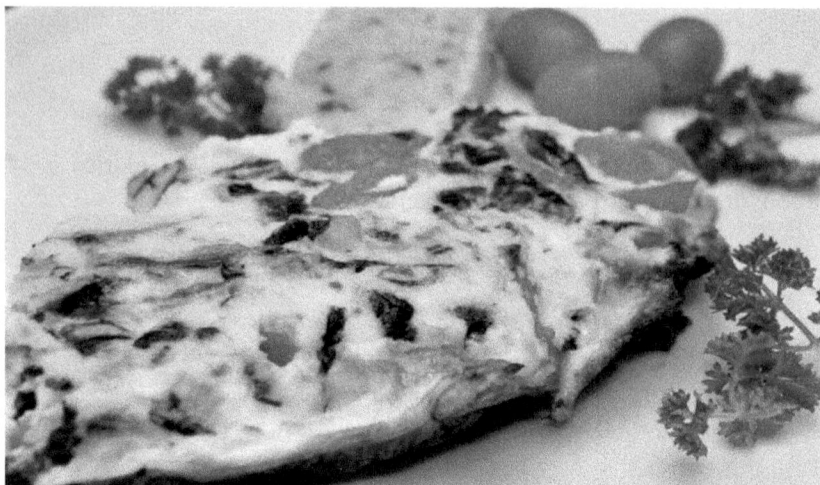

Ingredients

- 1 (pack) cup Baby spinach, stems removed and chopped

- 3 Whole eggs

- 3 Egg whites

- 1 cup 2% Shredded mozzarella cheese, divided

- 2 tbsp. 1% milk

- ½ cup Onion, diced

- 1 Roma tomato, diced

- 1 tbsp. Extra virgin olive oil

- ¼ tsp. White pepper

- ¼ tsp. Black pepper

- Salt

Directions

1. Sauté onions on medium heat for about 5 minutes or until tender.

2. Lightly grease the crock with cooking spray.

3. In a large mixing bowl, mix the sautéed onions, ¾ cup mozzarella, and the rest of the ingredients. Whisk to combine and pour the mixture to the cooker. Top it with a quarter cup of mozzarella cheese.

4. Cover the slow cooker with lid and cook on low for about 1- 1 ½ hours or until the eggs are firm. Use the toothpick pick test to make sure that the frittata is done.

Serving: **6**

Nutritional Facts (⅙ of the recipe): Calories - 139; Carbohydrates - 4g; Fats - 8g; Protein - 12g

Slow Cooker Baked Apples

Ingredients

- 1 ¼ cups Granola
- 5 Medium gala apples
- tbsp. Grass-fed butter, melted
- tsp. Maple syrup

Directions

1. Cut off the top of the apples with a knife. Using a melon baller tool or a metal measuring teaspoon, remove the core (including the seeds) from each apple.

2. Put ¼ cup granola into each apple and put them into the cooker.

3. Drizzle the apples with butter and to each, a teaspoon of maple syrup.

4. Cover the cooker with lid and cook on high for about 2 ½ to 3 hours or until the apples are tender yet firm.

Serving: 5

Nutritional Facts: Calories - 313; Carbohydrates - 48g; Fats - 12g; Protein - 4g

Slow Cooker Banana French Toast

Ingredients

- 1 x 10-inch French baguette (1 to 2-day old), cut into 1-inch slices

- 4 bananas, sliced into rounds

- 3 eggs, lightly whisked

- 4 oz. Cream cheese, softened at room temperature

- ½ cup Walnuts or pecans, chopped

- ¼ cup Skim milk

- 2 tbsp. Light brown sugar

- ⅓ cup Honey (plus more to drizzle)

- 1 tsp. Ground cinnamon

- Pinch of nutmeg

- ½ tbsp. Pure vanilla extract

- 2 tbsp. Butter, cut into thin slices

Directions

1. Coat the crock of your cooker with nonstick cooking spray.

2. Apply cream cheese of on both sides of each bread slice. Assemble the slices at the bottom of the crock.

3. Put the banana slices on top of the bread. Sprinkle with nuts and sugar. Put the butter slices on top and set aside.

4. Add the honey, vanilla extract, milk, nutmeg, and cinnamon with eggs. Whisk until well combined. Pour the mixture over the bread. (Note: The egg mixture shouldn't only coat the bread but should come up about ¾ to the brim. If it's less, add more egg mixture.)

5. Cover with lid and cook for about 3-4 hours on low (or 2-2 ½ hrs. on high). After that, remove the lid and switch to the "warm" setting.

6. Transfer to serving plates and drizzle the toast slices with honey before serving.

Serving: 6

Nutritional Facts (2 slices per serving): Calories - 438; Carbohydrates - 56g; Fats - 20g; Protein - 10g

Slow Cooker Brown Rice Chicken Congee

Ingredients

- 1 cup Brown rice
- 1 Skinless chicken breast
- cups Low-sodium chicken broth
- cups Water
- 3 tbsp. Soy sauce
- 2 tbsp. Ginger, grated
- 1 clove Garlic, peeled and smashed
- 1 tbsp. Lime juice
- 2 tbsp. Sesame oil
- 1 tsp. Hot chili flakes
- ¼ tsp. Salt

For the toppings:

- Green onions, sliced
- Peanuts, chopped
- Cilantro, chopped
- Sesame oil

Directions

1   Put the rice, chicken, water, broth, garlic, ginger, soy sauce, chili flakes, and salt to the cooker.

2   Set the cooker on low and cook for about 8 hours (or on high for about 4 hours).

3   Once done, stir the congee (if needed, add more water to adjust the consistency) and remove the chicken. Shred the chicken, discarding the bones if there are, and return to the congee.

4   Stir in the lime juice and sesame oil. Serve with favorite toppings.

Serving: 6

Nutritional Facts: Calories - 257; Carbohydrates - 26.3g; Fats -10.3g; Protein - 14.6g

Slow-Cooker Cobbler

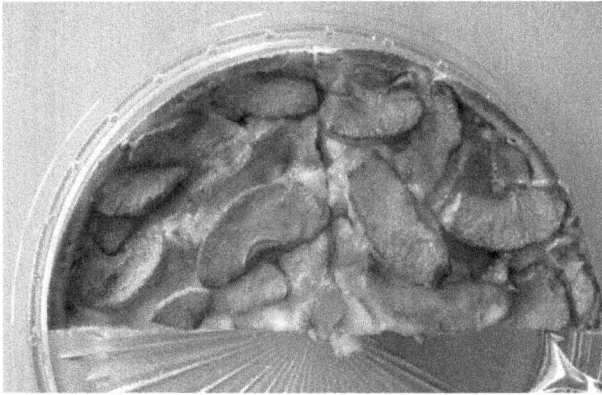

Ingredients

- 2 cups Granola cereal
- 3 cups Tart apples, peeled and sliced
- ¼ cup Honey
- 3 tbsp. Grass-fed butter, melted
- 1 tsp. Cinnamon

Directions

1. Lightly grease the crock with a nonstick cooking spray.

2. Layer the apples at the bottom of the crock. Sprinkle the apples with cinnamon and granola.

3. In a small mixing bowl, combine the butter and honey together. Mix well to make sure they're well combined.

4. Pour the honey-butter mixture over the apples and mix to coat well.

5. Cover the slow cooker with lid and set on low. Cook for about 5-7 hours or until the apples are fork-tender. Serve with homemade yogurt if desired.

Serving: 4

Nutritional Facts: Calories - 246; Carbohydrates - 44g; Fats - 9g; Protein - 1g

Slow-Cooker Maple-Glazed Squash

Ingredients

- 1 x 3-lb. Butternut
- tbsp. Maple sugar
- ¼ tsp. Ground cinnamon
- 1 tbsp. Unsalted butter, at room temperature
- Pinch of nutmeg, freshly grated
- Pinch of ground allspice
- ½ tsp. Kosher salt

For serving:

- Fruit, chopped
- Homemade yogurt
- Granola

Directions

1   Line the bottom of the crock with an aluminum foil, making sure it comes up on the sides as this will serve as your handle later on. Smear butter over the foil.

2   Cut the butternut into 8 wedges. Scoop out its seedy core and discard.

3   Mix the cinnamon, maple sugar, allspice, nutmeg, and salt in a bowl.

4   Lightly coat each squash wedge with the maple sugar mixture, arranging each with skin-side down at the foil-lined bottom of the slow cooker. Make sure you only make a single layer of these

squash wedges. Sprinkle excess maple sugar mixture over the squash wedges.

5   Cover the cooker with lid and cook on low for about 4-6 hours or until the squash is tender but not falling apart.

6   Transfer the wedges to a platter. Lift the corners of the foil and pour the juices over the squash wedges.

7   Serve with granola, chopped fruits, and/or homemade yogurt. If you have leftovers, store them in an airtight container and refrigerate for up to 4-5 days.

Serving: 8

Nutritional Facts: Calories - 89; Carbohydrates - 19.9g; Fats - 1.6g; Protein - 1.5g

Slow Cooker Overnight Carrot Cake Oatmeal

Ingredients

- 1 cup Steel-cut oats
- 1 cup Carrots, shredded
- ¾ cup Pineapple, chopped
- 4 cups Water
- ½ cup Grassmilk half and half
- ½ cup Raisins
- ⅓ cup Muscovado sugar
- 2 tsp. Vanilla extract
- 1 tsp. Ground cinnamon

For garnish:

- ½ cup Walnuts
- ¼ cup Coconut flakes, toasted

Directions

1. Add the oats, pineapple, raisins, muscovado sugar, carrots, half and half, cinnamon, and vanilla into the crock. Cover and set the cooker to low. Cook for 8 hours or overnight.

2. Stir the oatmeal and divide between serving bowls. Top each bowl with 1 tbsp. coconut flakes and 2 tbsp. walnuts.

Serving: 4

Nutritional Facts: Calories - 267; Carbohydrates - 47g; Fats - 10g; Protein - 7g

Slow Cooker Peach Oatmeal

Ingredients

- 1 cup Dry old-fashioned oats

- 1 cup Canned peaches in light syrup, diced

- ½ cup Walnuts (or pecans), chopped

- 2 cups Grass-fed milk

- 1 tbsp. Grass-fed butter

- 4-5 tbsp. Honey

- ½ tsp. Cinnamon

- ¼ tsp. Salt

Directions

1   Spray the crock of the slow cooker with a nonstick cooking spray.

2   In a mixing bowl, add all the ingredients and stir lightly.

3   Pour the mixture into the cooker. Cover the cooker with lid and cook on low for about 4 hours. Once done, the pats should be soft.

4   If desired, pour extra milk on top of the oatmeal. Serve and enjoy!

Serving: 4

Nutritional Facts: Calories - 325; Carbohydrates - 50g; Fats - 12g; Protein - 8.7g

Slow-Cooker Veggie Omelet

Ingredients

- Slow-Cooker Veggie Omelet
- Ingredients
- 1 cup Broccoli florets
- 6 Eggs
- 1 Red bell pepper, thinly sliced
- ½ cup Milk
- 1 Small yellow onion, finely chopped
- 1 Garlic clove, minced
- ⅛ tsp. Garlic powder
- ⅛ tsp. Chili powder
- ¼ tsp. Salt
- Fresh ground pepper

For garnish:

- Organic cheddar cheese, shredded
- Tomatoes, chopped
- Onions, chopped
- Fresh parsley

Directions

1. Lightly coat the crock with nonstick cooking spray then set aside.

2. Whisk the eggs, milk, chili powder, garlic powder, salt, and black pepper in a large mixing bowl until completely incorporated.

3. Put in the broccoli, onions, peppers, and garlic to the cooker. Add the egg mixture and stir well.

4. Set cooker on high and cook for 1 ½ to 2 hours or until the eggs are set.

5. Sprinkle with cheddar and cover with lid. Let stand for about 2-3 minutes or until the cheese has melted, then turn the slow cooker off.

6. Divide into 8 wedges. Serve with onions, tomatoes, and parsley as the choice of toppings.

Serving: 4

Nutritional Facts: Calories - 142; Carbohydrates - 8g; Fats - 7g; Protein - 10g

Lunch

Beef Tacos with Green Sauce

Ingredients

- 1 tbsp. Olive oil
- 1 3-lb. Boneless beef chuck roast
- 1/2 tsp. Ground cumin
- Kosher salt
- Freshly ground pepper
- 1 16-oz. jar salsa Verde
- 1/2 white onion, thinly sliced
- 2 cloves garlic, minced
- 1/2 cup Fresh cilantro, chopped
- 12 whole wheat tortillas, warmed

For toppings:

- Shredded lettuce and chopped tomatoes,
- Avocado and/or radishes,
- Lime wedges, for garnish

Directions

1. Preheat skillet and add olive oil over medium-high heat.

2. Season meat with pepper, salt, and cumin and add to the skillet. Cook until golden brown. Flip and cook for another 3 minutes. Do this to the rest of the meat.

3. Transfer the dish to the slow cooker, adding onion, garlic, and salsa. Secure over and set cooking for 6 hours on high.

4. Transfer meat to a platter or shallow pan and shred into pieces using two forks while discarding excess fat. Return shredded meat into the slow cooker, stirring in the cilantro.

5. Serve dish on in tortillas with desired toppings. Garnish with lime wedges.

Serving: 6

Nutritional Facts: Calories - 728; Carbohydrates - 44.35g; Fats - 30.36 g; Protein - 69.67 g

Butter Bean Minestrone

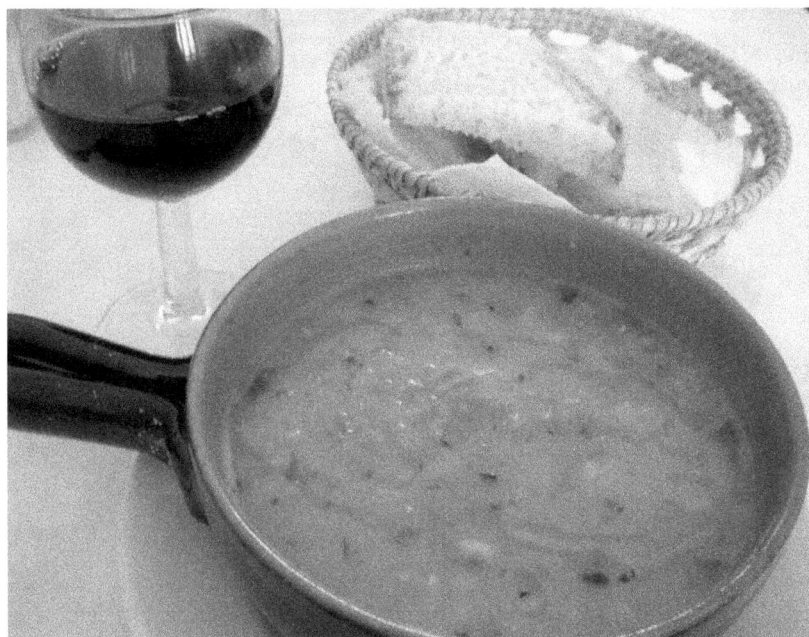

Ingredients

For the minestrone:

- 1 lb. Dried butter beans
- 1 Small zucchini, diced
- Medium plum tomatoes, diced
- 1 Large carrot, diced
- 2 Medium sweet onions, diced
- ¼ cup Extra-virgin olive oil, divided
- 2 qt. Low-sodium vegetable (or chicken broth)
- 1 Celery stalk, diced

- 1 tsp. Fennel seeds, freshly ground

- 1 tsp. Black pepper, freshly ground

- Kosher salt

For the basil pistou:

- cups Lightly packed fresh basil leaves

- ½ cup Parmigiano-Reggiano cheese, grated

- ½ cup Unsalted pistachios, shelled and roasted

- ½ cup Olive oil

- Kosher salt

- Freshly ground black pepper

Directions

1. In a large bowl, put the beans and soak them in water. Make sure that the water covers the beans by 3 inches. Refrigerate it overnight.

2. The next day, heat 2 tbsp. olive oil in skillet and sauté onions for about 5 minutes or until soft.

3. Drain and rinse the beans then put them into the cooker. Add the sautéed onions, celery, carrots and broth. Cover the cooker with lid and cook on low for about 6-8 hours or until tender.

4. Meanwhile, make the basil pistou by filling a large saucepan with water and bringing it to a boil. Add water into a large bowl and put some ice cubes. Put it nearby.

5. Add a tablespoon salt to the boiling water. Blanch the basil for about 20 seconds or until it begins to have a bright green color.

6. Using a slotted spoon, remove the basil from the boiling water and give it an ice bath. Strain the basil and wrap it in a kitchen towel. Squeeze gently to eliminate excess liquid.

7. Put the Parmigiano-Reggiano, blanched basil, and pistachios into a food processor. Start to process the contents, adding small amounts of olive oil until a paste is achieved. Season with salt and pepper if desired. Transfer into a serving bowl, cover with a plastic wrap and

refrigerate.

8   To finalize the minestrone, add the tomatoes, pepper, zucchini, fennel, and a tablespoon salt into the beans. Mix well to combine. Cover the cooker again and cook for another hour. Add salt if desired.

9   To serve, ladle into bowls and garnish each with basil pistou. Drizzle with olive oil and serve.

Serving: 6

Nutritional Facts: Calories - 596; Carbohydrates - 43.2g; Fats - 39.8g; Protein - 19.8g

Cauliflower Bolognese with Zucchini Noodles

Ingredients

For the bolognese:

- 1 Large cauliflower head cut up into florets
- 2 x 14-oz. cans Diced tomatoes
- ¾ cup diced red onion
- ½ cup Low-sodium vegetable broth
- 2 cloves Garlic, minced
- 2 tsp. Dried oregano flakes
- 1 tsp. Dried basil flakes
- ¼ tsp. Red pepper flakes
- Salt
- Black pepper

For the pasta:

- 5 large zucchinis, spiraled using Blade A

Directions

1. Put all the bolognese ingredients into the slow cooker. Cook on high for about 3 ½ hours.

2. Once done, mash the cauliflower florets using a fork or potato masher to make a "bolognese" consistency.

3. Divide zucchini noodles into bowls and ladle the bolognese over the noodles.

Serving: **6**

Nutritional Facts: Calories - 82; Carbohydrates - 16.71g; Fats - 1g; Protein - 4.88g

Citrusy Chipotle-Shrimp in Lettuce Cups

Ingredients

- 2 lb. Medium shrimp, peeled and deveined
- 4 Oranges
- 1 bunch Asparagus, trimmed and divided into three parts
- 16 Butter lettuce leaves
- 1 x 28-oz. can Diced tomatoes
- 2 Avocados, peeled, pitted, and diced
- 2 tbsp. Chipotle chilies in adobo, chopped
- 2 tbsp. Coconut oil
- ¼ cup Fresh flat-leaf parsley, chopped
- 2 tbsp. Tomato paste
- 1 tsp. Red pepper flakes

Directions

1. Get the zest from the oranges and set aside.

2. Peel off the remaining orange skins and discard them.

3. Working over a large bowl, hold the fruit on your non-dominant hand and the knife on the dominant one. Slice through the membranes, allowing them to drop into the bowl. Continue to do this step until you done with the oranges. Set aside.

4. Place the tomatoes, asparagus, shrimp, chipotles, tomato paste, orange zest, red pepper flakes, and coconut oil into the crock and toss to combine.

5. Put the crock back to the unit and cover with lid. Cook on low for 1 ½ hours. Make sure that the shrimp is no longer translucent.

6. Once done, arrange the lettuce on a platter. Spoon the shrimp-veggie mixture onto the lettuce and garnish with orange, avocado, and parsley. Serve.

Serving: 8

Nutritional Facts: Calories - 310; Carbohydrates - 24g; Fats - 12g; Protein - 27g

Japanese-Style Slow Cooker Tofu

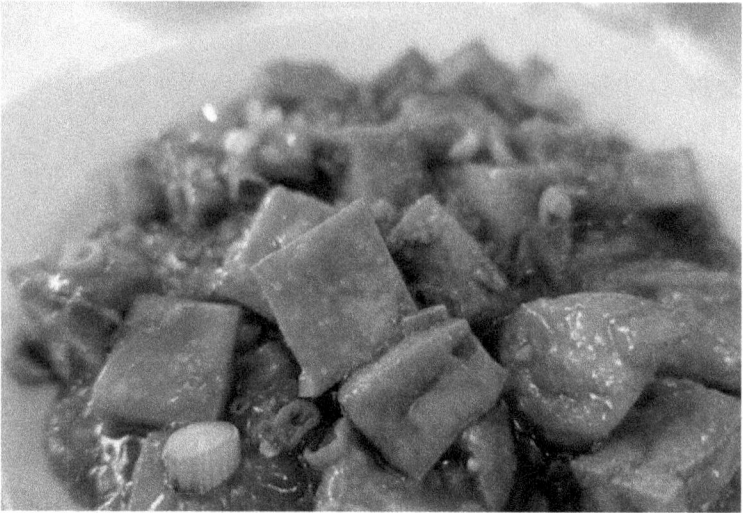

Ingredients

- 1 lb. Extra-firm tofu, drained and cut into ½-inch slices

- 1 bunch Fresh spinach leaves

- ¼ cup White miso paste

- ¼ cup Tamari

- 1 tbsp. Agave

- tbsp. Sesame oil

- tbsp. Water

- tbsp. Organic peanut butter

- 1 Green onion, thinly sliced

- 2 tbsp. Sesame seeds, toasted

Directions

1   Mix the tamari, peanut butter, miso, sesame oil, honey, and water in a medium-sized bowl.

2   Dip each tofu slice into the sauce to coat and layering them at the bottom of the cooker as you work.

3   Pour the remaining sauce over the tofu. Cover the cooker with lid and cook on low for about 4 hours or until the tofu is heated all the way through.

4   Add the spinach to the cooker and cook for about 10 minutes more.

5   Carefully spoon the some and tofu slices from the cooker to serving plates. Garnish each serving with green onions and sesame seeds. Serve and enjoy!

Serving: 4

Nutritional Facts: Calories - 281; Carbohydrates - 14.3g; Fats - 18.7g; Protein - 19g

Korean Gochujang Pork

Ingredients

- lb. Pork shoulder or butt

- ⅓ cup Gochujang

- ¼ cup Low-sodium soy sauce

- ¼ cup Honey

- ½ cup Chicken stock

Directions

1   Place the pork shoulder at the bottom of the slow cooker.

2   In a mixing bowl, whisk the honey, gochujang, stock, and soy sauce. Pour over the pork. Cover the cooker with lid and cook on low for about 8-10 hours.

3   Once done, transfer the pork into a large bowl and the juices into a sauce pan. Let it boil for about 15-20 minutes or until it diminishes to about 2 cups.

4   Meanwhile, shred the pork using two forks. Pull it across the grain to attain long strands of meat instead of short chunks.

5   Once the sauce is done, pour it over the shredded pork and toss to coat.

Serving: 12

Nutritional Facts: Calories - 491; Carbohydrates - 10.6g; Fats - 34.2g; Protein - 33.2g

Pinto Beans, Tomatoes and Onion Salad

Ingredients

- 3 cups Dried pinto beans, soaked overnight or for at least 6 hours

- 1 big red onion, sliced

- 2 cups Cherry tomatoes, halved (or 3 big tomatoes, diced)

- 3 sprigs Fresh parsley

- 8 cups Water

- 3 tbsp. Extra virgin olive oil

- 1 ¼ tsp. Salt

- ¼ tsp. Ground black pepper

Directions

1. Drain and discard the water where you soaked the beans.

2. Add the beans, water, salt, and pepper to the slow cooker. Cook on high for about 6 hours.

3. Drain and discard the water then transfer the beans to a serving bowl. Add the tomatoes and onions then mix everything.

4. Drizzle with olive oil. Sprinkle with parsley and salt before serving.

Serving: 8

Nutritional Facts: Calories - 313; Carbohydrates - 49g; Fats - 6g; Protein - 16g

Potato- Cauliflower Curry

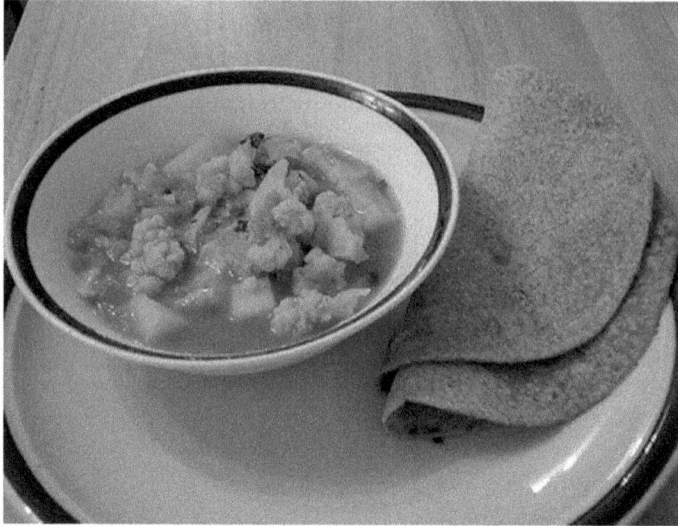

Ingredients

- 2 cups low sodium veggie broth

- 2 -14 oz. cans coconut milk

- 1/4 cup Thai Red curry paste

- 1 tbsp. Molasses (pomegranate or regular molasses)

- 1/2 tsp. Cumin seeds

- 2 cups Fresh spinach

- 1 lb. Baby potatoes, cut in halves

- 2 tbsp. Low-sodium soy sauce

- 1 Cinnamon stick

- 1 large Head cauliflower, cut into florets

- Kosher salt and pepper

For serving

- Steamed rice, cilantro, and limes

- Fresh Naan bread

- Arils from a pomegranate

Directions

1. Place coconut milk, curry paste, molasses, soy sauce and broth in the slow cooker.

2. Add cauliflower florets, potatoes, cumin, and cinnamon. Season it with salt and pepper to taste. Secure lid and cook for 3-4 hours on high or if you prefer to cook on low heat, cook for 5-6 hours.

3. Add spinach into the curry, stir, and cook for another 5 minutes until leaves are wilted.

4. Ladle into bowls topped with pomegranate arils, lime, and cilantro. Serve with fresh naan bread or rice.

Serving: 6

Nutritional Facts (per serving): Calories - 358; Carbohydrates -38 g; Fats- 55g; Protein - 7g

Quinoa Pilaf with Wild Rice

Ingredients

In the cooker:

- 1 ¼ cup Quinoa
- ¾ cup Wild rice
- 2 Golden beets, chopped
- ⅓ cup Shallot or red onion, chopped
- 1 cup Fresh cranberries
- 2 ¼- 3 cups broth
- 3 tbsp. Orange juice
- ½- 1 tsp. Dry herb season mix
- ½ tsp. Sea salt
- ½ tsp. Black pepper
- 1 cup Broccoli, chopped

To serve:

- 1 cup Feta crumble
- ½ cup Fresh basil or parsley
- ½ cup pumpkin or sunflower seeds, roasted
- Dried cranberries
- 1 tbsp. Olive oil
- Salt
- Black pepper

Directions

1. Put all the ingredients (except for the broccoli) into the cooker. Mix well to combine.

2. Cook on low for about 5 hours (or on high for 2- 2 ½ hours). Check halfway and mix with a spoon. If the pilaf is too dry, add ¼- ¾ cup of broth; if there's too much liquid, discard a few tablespoons of liquid and cook a bit longer.

3. Once done, the quinoa should be fluffy and the rice a little al dente. Transfer the contents to a large serving bowl. Add the "to serve" ingredients (except for the fresh basil or parsley), season with salt and pepper, and mix everything up. Top with fresh parsley or basil and serve.

Serving: 8 (serving size of ½ cup)

Nutritional Facts: Calories - 236; Carbohydrates - 32.3g; Fats - 8.3g; Protein - 9.2g

Slow Cooker Korean Chicken

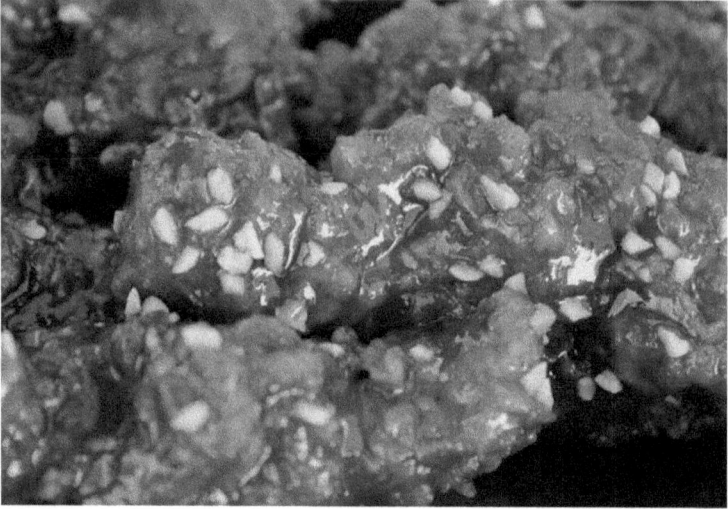

Ingredients

- 1 lb. Boneless and skinless chicken thighs, chopped

- 1 lb. Boneless and skinless chicken breast, chopped

- ⅓ cup Low-sodium soy sauce

- ⅓ cup honey

- Jalapenos, diced

- cloves Garlic, whole

- ½ Red onion, diced

- 1 tbsp. Fresh ginger, peeled and grated

- 2 tbsp. Sesame seeds

- 2 tbsp. Rice vinegar

Directions

1 In a small mixing bowl, combine the honey, soy sauce, rice vinegar, ginger, onion, jalapeños, and sesame seeds.

2 Line the chicken breasts and thighs to the slow cooker and cover with the honey-soy sauce mixture.

3 Cover the cooker with lid and cook on low for about 6-8 hours. Remove the lid in the last 30 minutes of cooking time to allow thickening of the sauce.

Serving: 8

Nutritional Facts: Calories - 197; Carbohydrates - 13g; Fats - 4g; Protein - 24g

Slow-Cooker Kung Pao Chickpeas

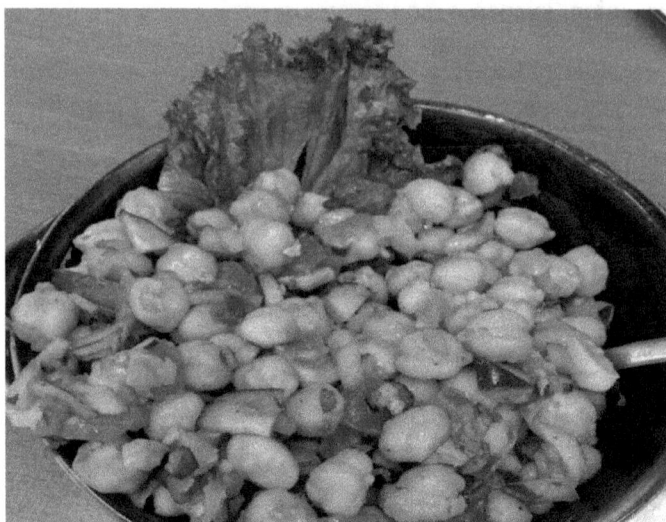

Ingredients

- ½ Red onion, chopped

- 1 Red bell pepper, chopped

- 2 x 15-oz. cans Chickpeas, rinsed and drained

- ¼ cup Tamari

- 2 tbsp. Balsamic vinegar

- 2 tbsp. Maple syrup

- ½ tsp. Garlic powder

- ½ tsp. Ground ginger

- 1 tsp. Red pepper flakes

- 1 tsp. Toasted sesame oil

- 3 Green onions, chopped

To serve:

- Sesame seeds (for garnish)

- Cauliflower rice (or brown rice)

Directions

1. Place the chickpeas, onion, and bell pepper into the cooker.

2. In a small mixing bowl, incorporate the maple syrup, tamari, ginger, sesame oil, vinegar, garlic, and red pepper flakes. Pour the mixture over the chickpea mixture and stir to combine.

3. Cover the cooker with lid and cook on low for about 6 hours (or on high for 3 hours). You can add 2-4 tablespoons of water to avoid overcooking the sauce.

4. Once done, stir the chickpeas and ladle over a bowl of cauliflower rice. You may garnish with green onions and sesame seeds when serving.

Serving: 6

Nutritional Facts: Calories - 120; Carbohydrates - 19g; Fats - 2g; Protein - 8g

Slow Cooker Mushroom Barley Risotto

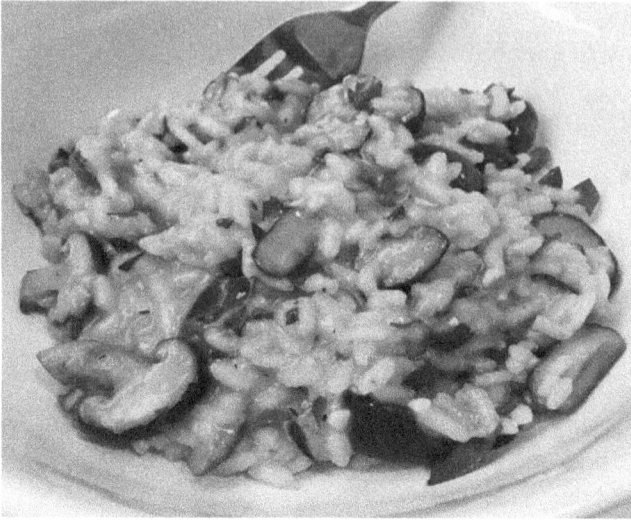

Ingredients

- 1 lb. Cremini mushrooms, sliced
- 3 cups Lower-sodium vegetable broth
- 1 ½ cups Pearl barley
- ¼ cup Fresh flat-leaf parsley, chopped
- ⅔ cup Organic parmesan, grated
- 2 tbsp. Extra-virgin olive oil
- 8 oz. Carrots, finely chopped
- 1 Large onion, finely chopped
- 4 sprigs Fresh Thyme
- 1 tbsp. Sherry vinegar
- Kosher salt
- Black pepper, freshly ground

Directions

1. Heat olive oil in a saucepan over medium-high heat before adding the onions plus ⅛ tsp. each of salt and pepper. Sauté for about 5 minutes or until lightly browned, stirring occasionally.

2. Add the mushrooms and continue to cook for about 2 minutes or until the mushrooms are browned. Stir occasionally to avoid burning.

3. Add the thyme and barley. Continue cooking for about 2 minutes, stirring occasionally until the barley is golden then turn off the heat.

4. Transfer the contents to the cooker. Add the carrots, ¼ tsp. salt, broth, and 1 ½ cups of water then cover the cooker with lid.

5. Cook on high for about 3 hours or until the liquid has been absorbed and the carrots and barley are tender.

6. Remove the thyme and discard. Mix in the parmesan, sherry vinegar, ½ tsp. salt, and ¼tsp. pepper. If needed, add warm water to thin out risotto into your preferred consistency.

7. To serve, garnish with parsley and/or season more with salt and pepper.

Serving: 4

Nutritional Facts: Calories - 435; Carbohydrates - 75g; Fats - 10g; Protein - 14g

Slow-Cooked Okra and Tomato

Ingredients

- 1 lb. Okra, sliced in ¾-inch pieces

- 1 Large tomato, diced

- 1 Onion, diced

- 1 x 8-oz.can of Sugar-free tomato sauce

- cloves garlic, diced

- 1 cup Water

- 2 tsp. Salt

- 1 tsp. Black pepper

Directions

1. Put all ingredients into the slow cooker and cook on medium setting for 4-6 hours or until the okra is soft. Remember to stir occasionally.

Serving: 4

Nutritional Facts: Calories - 74; Carbohydrates - 16.7g; Fats - 0.5g; Protein - 3.74g

Slow Cooker Roast Vegetables

Ingredients

- 3 Small zucchini, cut in thick slices

- 2 Bell peppers, cut in large slices

- 1 Large sweet potato, peeled and cubed

- 1 tsp. Italian seasoning

- ½ cup Garlic cloves, peeled

- 2 tbsp. Olive oil

- ½ tsp. Salt

Directions

1. Coat the crock with nonstick spray and put all the vegetables, garlic, salt, and oil. Toss to coat well.

2. Cook on low for 6 hours (or 3 hours on high), stirring once every hour. Open the lid and transfer the liquid to a clean container (Note: Do not discard. You can drink it or use it for other cooking purposes.)

Serving: 4

Nutritional Facts: Calories - 114; Carbohydrates - 18.4g; Fats - 4g; Protein - 3.9g

Slow Cooker Spanish Rice

Ingredients

- 1 cup Brown rice
- 1 x 4oz. can Diced green chilies
- ½ cup Tomatoes, diced
- ½ Jalapeno, de-seeded and diced
- 1 cup Chicken stock
- 1 cup Tomato sauce
- 1 tsp. Cumin
- ½ tsp. Chili powder
- ½ tsp. Dried oregano
- ½ tsp. Salt
- ¼ tsp. Pepper
- Fresh cilantro, to garnish
- Lime wedges, to garnish

Directions

1   Coat the crock of slow cooker with non-stick cooking spray.

2   Put the rice, stock, tomatoes, jalapeno, chilies, tomato sauce, oregano, cumin, chili powder, salt, and pepper into the cooker. Set the cooker on high. Cook for 2 ½ hours on high heat or for 5 hours on low.

3   Transfer to serving bowls. Garnish with cilantro and lime wedges.

Serving: 4

Nutritional Facts: Calories- 210; Carbohydrates- 44.2g; Fats- 1.8g; Protein- 5.4g

Slow Cooker Stuffed Peppers

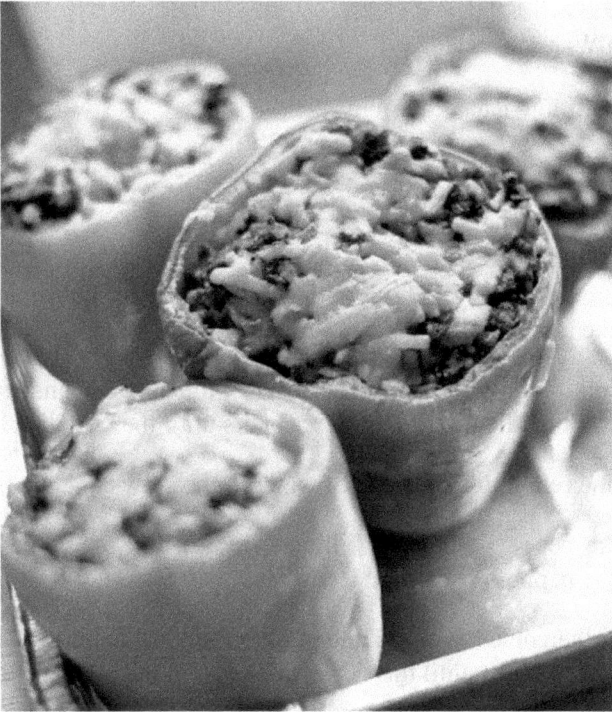

Ingredients

- 4 Large bell peppers, different colors

- 1 x 15-oz. can Black beans, drained and rinsed

- 1 x 14.5-oz can Fire-roasted diced tomatoes

- 1 cup Organic shredded cheese blend

- 1 tsp. Garlic powder

- 1 tsp. Cumin

- 1 tsp. Onion powder

- 3 tsp. Chili powder

- ½ tsp. Chipotle chili powder

- ½ tsp. Dried cilantro

- 1 cup Water, divided

- 1 cup Minute Rice Premium

Directions

1. Prepare large peppers by washing and cutting off their tops. Remove also the ribs and the seeds.

2. In a mixing bowl, incorporate the rice, tomatoes, beans, and half cup water. Stuff the mixture to the peppers until they're filled to the top.

3. Add the remaining half cup of water to the slow cooker.

4. Put the peppers (with the filling side up) into the cooker carefully. Top the peppers with cheese.

5. Cover the cooker with lid and cook on low for about 4-6 hours (or 2-3 hours on high) until the rice is cooked and the peppers are tender.

Serving: 4

Nutritional Facts: Calories - 345; Carbohydrates - 49g; Fats - 4g; Protein - 17g

Slow Cooker Turmeric Lentil Chili

Ingredients

- 1 cup Coconut milk in a can
- (15-oz) cans kidney beans, drained and rinsed
- 1 small yellow onion, finely chopped
- 32-oz reduced-sodium vegetable stock
- cups brown or green lentils
- 6-oz. can of Tomato paste
- Cilantro, chopped
- Green onion, chopped
- 1 tsp. Ground cumin
- 1 tsp. Chili powder
- 1 tsp. Turmeric
- 2 cups water
- 1 ½ tsp. Kosher salt
- Freshly Sliced avocado (for topping)

Directions

1   Add all ingredients into the slow cooker and cook on high for 6 hours on low or 4 hours on high. Then check if lentils are tender.

2   When done, add the coconut milk, stir to blend. If the consistency of the mixture is too dry, you may add stock or water and allow it to simmer until you achieve desired consistency.

3   Adjust seasoning to taste. Serve.

Serving: 6

Nutritional Facts: Calories - 418; Carbohydrates - 48.99 g; Fats - 89.2 g; Protein – 41.37 g

Sweet Potato Chipotle Chili

Ingredients

- 1 lb. Ground lean turkey
- 3 cups Riced cauliflower
- 4 cups Sweet potatoes, peeled and chopped
- 1 x 14-oz. Diced canned tomatoes, drained
- 1 cup White onion, chopped
- 2 cups Broth
- 1 tsp. Garlic, minced
- 2 Chipotles with the adobo sauce, chopped
- ½ cup Bell peppers, chopped
- 1 tsp. Cumin
- ½ tsp. Paprika
- ½ tsp. Chili powder
- ¼ tsp. Black pepper
- Sea salt

For garnish (optional):

- Cilantro, chopped
- Jalapeño, chopped

Directions

1. Put the potatoes in a microwave-safe bowl and steam with a tablespoon of water for about 1 ½ minutes.

2. Place a skillet over medium heat and brown the turkey. Drain the grease and put into the cooker.

3. Add the potato, tomatoes, riced cauliflower, onion, and broth. Mix them together to combine.

4. Put the chipotle, bell peppers, and seasonings. Stir again, cover, and cook for about 1-2 hours. Start checking after an hour.

Serving: 6 (serving size of 1 ½ cups)

Nutritional Facts: Calories- 221; Carbohydrates- 21.3g; Fats- 7g; Protein- 19.3g

Veggie-Collagen-Chili Dish

Ingredients

- 1 Pack of Low sodium veggie broth

- 1 Bottle Tomato Marinara (low sodium)

- 1 can Black beans (cooked)

- 1 can Kidney beans (cooked)

- 2 cup Carrots, chopped

- ½ cup Yellow onions, chopped

- 1 tsp. Cumin

- 1 tsp. Coriander

- A bunch of fresh cilantro, chopped

- 2 tbsp. Reduced Tamari Soy Sauce

- 1 tbsp. Chili powder

- 3 tbsp. Collagen powder

Direction

1. Add all ingredients in a slow cooker and cook for 8 hours on low heat.

Serving: 4

Nutritional Facts (per serving): Calories -174; Carbohydrates - 20.22 Fats - 2.78 Protein –5.43g

Dinner

Anti-Inflammatory Curry Rice Vegetable Bowl

Ingredients

- 1 cup Brown rice

- 1 cup Broccoli, finely chopped

- 2 cups Mushrooms, finely chopped

- 1½ cups Green cabbage, finely chopped

- 4 cups of Vegetable Broth

- 2 tbsp. Apple cider vinegar

- 1 tsp. curry powder

- ½ tsp. Garlic powder

- ¼ tsp. Dry Thyme

- 1 tsp. Himalayan Salt

- ½ tsp. Ground black pepper

Directions

1. Put all the ingredients to the cooker, cover with lid, and cook on low for 3-4 hours or until the liquids have been absorbed. Add more water or broth if needed. Fluff with fork or spoon before serving.

Serving: 4

Nutritional Facts: Calories - 286; Carbohydrates - 54g; Fats - 5g; Protein - 13g

Asian Lettuce Wraps

Ingredients

For the filling:

- 2 lb. Ground chicken breast
- 12 leaves Butterhead or iceberg lettuce
- 1 x 8oz. can Water chestnuts, drained and chopped
- 1 x 14.5 oz. can Reduced-sodium chicken broth
- 1 cup Carrots, shredded
- 1 cup Edamame
- 3 Green onions
- 4 tsp. Reduced sodium soy sauce
- 1 tbsp. Chinese style hot mustard
- 2 tsp. Reduced sodium teriyaki sauce
- 1 tsp. Rice vinegar
- 2 tbsp. Hoisin sauce
- ½ tsp. Ground black pepper

For dipping sauce:

- 1 tbsp. Creamy peanut butter
- ¼ cup Soy sauce
- ¼ cup Rice vinegar
- 1 tbsp. Water
- ½ tbsp. Sweet chili sauce

For toppings (optional):

- Asian chili sauce

- Sesame seeds

Directions

1. Cut the green onions, separating the white from the green, then slice the green part into slivers.

2. Put the chicken breasts, water chestnuts, edamame, carrots, white parts of the green onions, mustard, teriyaki sauce, soy sauce, vinegar, and pepper into the cooker. Pour the broth and close the cooker.

3. Cook on high for about 2- 2 ½ hours (or 4-5 hours on low).

4. Strain the mixture to remove excess moisture and shred the chicken. Add the green onion slivers and hoisin sauce.

5. Serve with lettuce leaves, dipping sauce, and toppings.

Serving: 6

Nutritional Facts: Calories -258; Carbohydrates - 13g; Fats - 4g; Protein - 40g

Black Bean, Quinoa, and Sweet Potato Stew

Ingredients

- 11-oz can of corn
- cups Sweet potatoes cubed
- 2/3 cup Uncooked quinoa
- 4-5 cups Stock
- 19 oz. can diced tomatoes including juices
- 1 cup Red onion diced
- 19- oz. can black beans drained and rinsed
- tbsp. Cumin
- 1 tbsp. Chili powder
- 1 tsp. salt

After Cooking

- tbsp. Lime juice
- Adjust seasoning to taste

Directions

1   Add in ingredients to a large slow cooker and cook for about 8 hours on low.

2   Add lime juice and adjust seasoning to taste, adding more salt if needed.

Servings: 6

Nutrition Facts: Calories – 294; Carbohydrates – 58g; Fat – 4g; Protein- 11g

Beef and Black Bean Stew

Ingredients

- 1 lb. Lean beef stew meat

- 2 Carrots, diced

- 4 cups Low-sodium beef broth

- 1 Medium onion, coarsely chopped

- 2 x 15 oz. cans Black beans, drained

- 1 large potato, cubed

- 2 tbsp. Chili powder

- 2 tsp. Cumin

- 2 Bay leaves

- 1 tbsp. Extra-virgin olive oil

- 1 tsp. Kosher or sea salt

- ½ tsp. Black pepper

Directions

1. Put all the ingredients to the cooker, cover with lid, and cook on high for 6-8 hours (or on low for 3-4 hours).

Serving: 6

Nutritional Facts: Calories - 388; Carbohydrates - 51g; Fats - 6g; Protein - 34g

Brussels Sprouts with Cranberries, Pecans, and Butternut

Ingredients

- 14-oz. cups Brussels sprouts halved

- 4 cups of butternut squash, cubed

- 1 red onion cut into large chunks

For Maple Cinnamon Sauce

- 1/4 cup maple syrup

- tbsp. apple cider vinegar

- 1 tsp. McCormick ground cinnamon

- 1/4 tsp. Ground nutmeg

- 1/2 tsp. salt

Minutes before serving

- A cup of fresh cranberries

- Half a cup of pecans

Directions

1   Throw in Butternut squash cuts, Brussels sprouts, and red onion into a large slow cooker. Toss lightly to combine and cook on high for 2-2 ½ hours. Check after two hours of cooking. Brussels sprouts must be soft but still chewable while the butternut is likewise tender but not mushy.

2   Just before serving the dish, add fresh cranberries and cook for 5 minutes more.

3   In another pot, add maple syrup, nutmeg, cinnamon, apple cider vinegar, and salt. Cook over low-medium heat and bring to boil stirring frequently. When sauce thickens, turn off heat and pour sauce over veggies. Toss to blend.

4   Sprinkle your dish with pecans to serve.

Notes:

- When not immediately serving, remove veggies out of the slow cooker and reserve the liquid. Just spoon over the liquid when serving. You may cook this recipe in half but set cooking on low for 21/2 – 3 hours.

Servings: 8

Nutrition Facts: Calories – 129; Carbohydrates – 22g; Fat – 5g; Protein – 2g

Chicken Cacciatore with Cremini Mushrooms

Ingredients

- 1 whole chicken, skinless (cut into 10 pieces)
- 1 tbsp. whole wheat flour
- 8-oz Cremini mushrooms, quartered
- 28-oz. can of whole peeled plum tomatoes in juice (drained and chopped
- 1/4 cup dry white wine
- 1 celery stalk, thinly sliced
- 1 small onion, halved and thinly sliced
- 1 sprig fresh rosemary or 1/2 teaspoon dried rosemary, crumbled
- Coarse salt and ground pepper

Directions

1   Prepare a 5-quart slow cooker and place all ingredients in it. Cover and cook for four hours on high setting. Avoid lifting the cover while it is still cooking so as not to affect the cooking time.

2   Discard rosemary twig before serving with a cup of healthy brown rice or whole-grain bread.

Serving: 4

Nutritional Facts (per serving): Calories - 379; Carbohydrates - 92.36g; Fats - 2.32 g; Protein – 8.16 g

Easy Slow-Cooker Vegetable Korma

Ingredients

- 1 large cauliflower, cut into florets
- Large carrots, chopped
- 1/2 cup Frozen green peas 1 cup green beans, chopped
- 1/2 Onion, chopped
- 1 tsp. garam marsala
- 2 tbsp. Curry powder
- 2 tbsp. Red pepper flakes
- 2 cloves Garlic, minced
- 3/4 can of coconut milk
- 2 tbsp. almond meal
- Salt

Directions

1   Combine cauliflower florets, green peas, carrots, green beans, garlic, and onions in a large slow cooker. Arrange in layers with peas and beans on the floor of the cooker.

2   Once vegetables are done, in a large mixing bowl, mix coconut milk with garam marsala, curry powder, red pepper flakes, and sea salt. Toss thoroughly to mix well. Pour liquid mixture over cooked vegetables and sprinkle it with almond meal.

3   Continue cooking on low for 8 hours on low and 5 hours on high until the mixture thickens,

4   You can serve the dish hot or warm. Note that this dish tastes better when it sits longer. You can store it in the fridge for up to a week and in the freezer for up to two months.

Serving: 4

Nutritional Facts (per serving): Calories - 202; Carbohydrates - 22.11g; Fats - 12.21 g; Protein - 6.82 g

Beef Meatballs - Lebanese Green Beans

Ingredients

For the Beef Meatballs:

- 1/2 teaspoon cumin

- 1/4 teaspoon cayenne pepper

- 1/8 teaspoon black pepper

- 1/2 tsp. cinnamon

- 1/4 cup plain breadcrumbs from whole wheat bread

- 1 lb. ground beef

- 1/2 tsp. allspice

- 1/4 cup parsley, minced

- 1 tbsp. olive oil

- 1 tsp. salt

For the Lebanese Green Beans:

- 14.5-oz. cans of diced tomatoes

- 14.5 oz. can of tomato sauce

- 1 tsp. cumin

- 1 tsp. cinnamon

- 1/4 tsp. Cayenne pepper

- Salt and pepper to taste

- 1 lb. Green beans

- 1/2 Sweet onion, diced

- 2 Garlic cloves, minced

Directions

1   Divide cumin, cayenne pepper, cinnamon, pepper, and salt into two portions and set aside.

2   Add diced tomatoes with tomato sauce, cinnamon, cumin, cayenne pepper in the slow cooker and season with salt and pepper. Also, add green beans, garlic, and onions and mix well to blend.

3   In a mixing bowl, combine all remaining ingredients. Using your hands, use hands in mixing and rubbing mixture to the beef. When completely blended, form meatballs about an inch in diameter and arrange them at the bottom of the slow cooker, completely submerge in tomato sauce.

4   Cook in high setting for 4 hours or 8 hours on low setting.

5   Garnish with fresh parsley and serve with rice or pita bread.

Serving: 4

Nutritional Facts (per serving): Calories - 514.75; Carbohydrates - 38.67g; Fats - 23.18 g; Protein – 35.28 g

Greek Stuffed Peppers

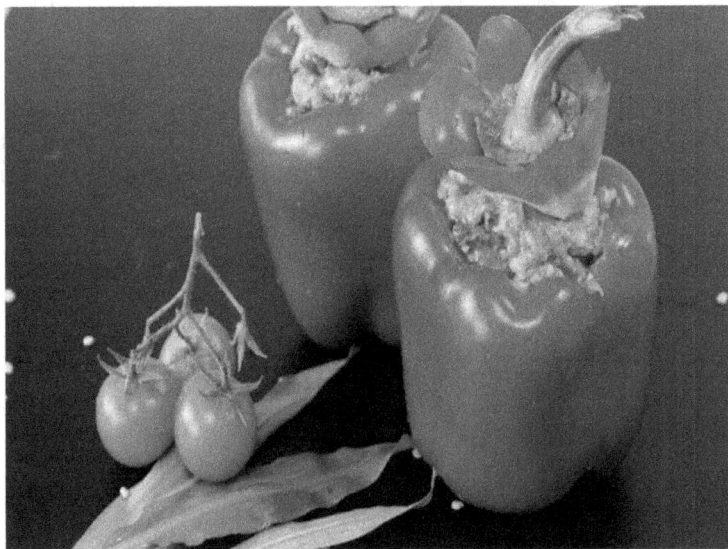

Ingredients

- 15-oz. can of cannellini beans, drained

- large bell peppers

- 1 cup crumbled feta

- scallions, julienned(separate white from green parts)

- 1/2 cup whole wheat couscous

- 1 garlic clove, minced

- Coarse salt

- Freshly ground pepper

- 1 tsp. Dried oregano

- Lemon wedges, for serving

Directions

1   Cut a thin slice on the bottom of bell peppers to allow them to stand. Cut off tops slightly just below the stem. Discard stem and clean the inside of each pepper, removing seeds.

2   Add all ingredients in a mixing bowl and toss to blend. Add salt and pepper for seasoning and stuff bell peppers. Arrange stuffed peppers inside the slow cooker in an upright position. Secure the lid cover and cook for 4 hours on high setting.

3   When done, arrange nicely on a large platter and garnish with lemon wedges.

Servings: 4

Nutritional Facts (per serving):

Slow-Cooker Lamb with Olives and Potatoes

Ingredients

- lbs. Lamb shanks, cut crosswise into (1.5 inches a piece)

- 1 1/4 lbs. Small potatoes, cut in halves

- tbsp. Almond Flour

- Large Shallots, cut into wedges (about half inch)

- tbsp. Lemon extract

- Cloves garlic, minced

- 1 tbsp. Grate lemon zest

- 3/4 cups Low-sodium chicken broth

- Sprigs of rosemary

- tbsp. Extra virgin olive oil

- 1/2 cup Dry white wine

- 1 cup of green olives, pitted and cut into halves

Directions

1   Add Garlic, shallots, potatoes, rosemary, and lemon zest in the slow cooker. Season with salt and pepper.

2   In a small mixing bowl, add a tablespoon of almond flour and broth. Mix and whisk before adding to the slow cooker.

3   Add the remaining 3 tablespoons of the almond flour on a plate.

4   Season lamb meat with salt and pepper and dip it in flour to coat. Shake to remove flour that didn't stick to the meat.

5   Preheat a large skillet and heat oil over medium-high heat. Cook meat in batches until all sides are brown before transferring to the slow cooker.

6   Add wine to the remaining meat juice on the skillet and cook, stirring to remove bits sticking to its bottom. Continue cooking until the liquid volume is reduced in half before adding to the slow cooker.

7   Cover slow cooker and set to cook for 7 hours on low or 3 ½ hours on high. After the allotted time, add olives, stir and continue cooking for 20 minutes more.

8   Once done, transfer dish to a platter. Serve with sauce taken from remaining cooking liquid and added with lemon juice.

Servings: 4

Nutritional Facts (per serving): Calories - 313; Carbohydrates - 26.47g; Fats - 23.18 g; Protein - 31.91g

Lebanese Green Beans - Beef

Ingredients

- 1 lb. Beef stew meat (cubed)

- 1 lb. Green beans, trimmed and cut in 2-inch a piece

- 32-oz. Tomatoes, crushed

- 1 tbsp. Cinnamon

- 1 Onion (medium) diced

- ¼ cup Parsley, chopped

- ½ tsp. Pepper

- ½ tbsp. Sea salt

- Cooked rice or pita bread to serve

Directions

1   Put in the slow cooker the beef, tomatoes, onions, and green beans.

2   Add cinnamon, season with salt and pepper and stir to blend.

3   Set cooking for 8 hours on low and for 4 hours on high.

4   Serve with rice or Pita bread.

Serving: 4

Nutritional Facts (per serving): Calories - 271; Carbohydrates -26.7 g; Fats- 4.8g; Protein - 30.9g

Moroccan Chicken and Squash

Ingredients

- 8-oz. Butternut squash, peeled and cut into chunks
- 1 tsp. ground cumin
- 2 tbsp. Tomato paste
- 1 Large turnip, peeled and chopped
- 3 cups Low Sodium Chicken broth
- 1/3 cup Raisins
- 3-4 lbs. Chicken legs
- 1 Leek1/2 tsp. Turmeric
- 1 tsp. Ground coriander
- Freshly ground pepper
- Kosher salt
- Grated zest and juice extract of a lemon
- Fresh cilantro (for topping)

Directions

1. Put squash, turnip, raisin, and leek in the slow cooker. Season chicken with salt and pepper. Lay it on top of vegetables.

2. In a large mixing bowl, combine chicken broth, cumin, tomato paste, turmeric, lemon zest and juice, coriander and a teaspoon of salt. Whisk and pour mixture over chicken and veggies. Secure cover and cook for 4 hours on high.

3. Serve drizzled with remaining liquid in the pot and top with cilantro.

Serving: 4

Nutritional Facts (per serving): Calories - 562; Carbohydrates - 15.91g; Fats - 18.16 g; Protein – 81.41g

Ratatouille

Ingredients

- 28-oz. Diced tomatoes, undrained
- 1 eggplant cut to half-inch a piece
- zucchini cut to half-inch a piece
- 2 yellow squash cut to half-inch a piece
- 1 red pepper, diced
- 1 onion, diced
- 1 tbsp. minced garlic
- 1 1/2 tsp. sea salt
- 1 tbsp. Italian seasoning
- 1/4 tsp. crushed red pepper
- 1/4 tsp. fresh ground black pepper
- 1 tsp. tomato paste
- 1 tbsp. Fresh parsley, chopped (alternative: chives)

Directions

1 Add tomatoes, zucchini, eggplant, squash, red pepper, Italian seasoning, onion, garlic, red pepper, black pepper, and salt in a slow cooker and cook on either 3 ½ hours for high heat setting and 6-8 hours on low.

2 Add parsley and tomato paste and continue cooking uncovered for about 30 minutes more.

3 Serve on a platter drizzled with olive oil if desired along with parsley or chives.

Serving: 6

Nutritional Facts (per serving): Calories - 86; Carbohydrates - 18.64g; Fats - 0.86 g; Protein – 4.11g

Rosemary – Carrot - Parsnip Mash

Ingredients

- Large carrots
- 1 tbsp. Olive oil
- 1 cup Almond milk
- 1/2 tsp. Minced garlic
- tbsp. Coconut oil
- Fresh rosemary sprigs
- 1/4 cup Coconut cream
- Large parsnips
- 1/4 tsp. Sea salt
- Black pepper
- Parmesan or rosemary sprigs for garnish

Directions

1   Cleansed all vegetables and peel when desired but not necessary.

2   Steam carrots and parsnips in a steamer or in the microwave for about 90 seconds.

3   Chop into smaller pieces and place on the slow cooker along with the almond milk, ¼ garlic, coconut oil, rosemary sprigs, and salt. Cover and cook on high

4   After an hour, skim milk on the sides that has turned brown in color and mash it up with vegetables. Continue cooking for 90 minutes more and be on lookout for browning on sides. After 2 ½ hours cooking on high heat, adjust setting to low while removing stick sprigs, leaving leaves that fell off.

5   Add coconut oil, ¼ tsp. of garlic (remaining, black pepper, and sea salt. Mash all ingredients until chunky.

6   Serve with extra rosemary and parmesan for garnish.

Servings: 4

Nutritional Facts (per serving): Calories -256; Carbohydrates – 33g; Fat - 14g; Protein 3g

Slow Cooker Eggplant Parmesan

Ingredients

- 2 Large (estimated 2 lb.) eggplants, peeled and cut into ⅓-inch rounds
- 3 Large eggs, lightly whisked
- 2 cups Mozzarella, shredded
- 1 ¼ cups Marinara sauce
- 1 ½ cups Seasoned bread crumbs
- ¼ cup Fresh basil, chopped
- Salt

Directions

1. Season the eggplant on both sides with salt, lining them up on paper towels. Leave it Set for 20 minutes before rinsing. Pat to dry.

2. Coat the crock of the slow cooker with nonstick cooking spray. Spread a quarter cup of marinara sauce on the bottom.

3. Prepare the eggplant slices by dipping each in egg and coating with bread crumbs. Assemble a layer over the sauce, topping it with a quarter cup of marinara and half a cup of shredded mozzarella. Continue to layer sauce, eggplant, and cheese (making about 4 layers). End with cheese on top, filling the cooker for at least ⅔ full.

4. Cover the cooker with lid and cook on low for 4-6 hours or until the eggplant is soft and the mozzarella has melted.

5. Transfer to the plates and sprinkle with basil before serving.

Serving: 6

Nutritional Facts: Calories - 345; Carbohydrates - 36g; Fats - 14g; Protein - 20g

Slow Cooker Enchilada Quinoa Bake

Ingredients

- 14.5-oz can Tomatoes with green chilies, undrained
- 14.5-oz can Pinto beans, drained and rinsed
- 14.5-oz can Black beans, drained and rinsed
- 1 x 8-oz. can Tomato sauce
- 2 ¼ cups Vegetable Broth
- 1 ½ cups Frozen corn
- 1 ½ cups Grass-fed cheddar
- 1 ¼ cups Yellow onion, chopped
- 1 ¼ cups Red bell pepper, chopped
- 1 ½ cups Dry quinoa
- 2 tbsp. Chili powder
- 1 ½ tsp. Ground cumin
- 3 cloves Garlic, minced
- 1 tbsp. Canola oil
- Salt
- Black pepper, freshly ground

To serve:

- Roma tomatoes, diced

- Avocados, diced

- Cilantro, chopped

- Lime wedges,

- Green onions, chopped

Directions

1. Put the skillet over medium-high heat and add canola oil. Sauté the bell peppers and onions for 3 minutes before adding the garlic. Continue cooking for about 30 seconds more. Transfer the mixture into the cooker.

2. Add the tomatoes, tomato sauce, quinoa, cumin, and chili powder. Stir in the broth then season with salt and pepper.

3. Cover the cooker with lid and set on high for 2 hours and 45 minutes to 3 hours and 15 minutes. Monitor it to make sure that it's neither dry nor soggy.

4. Add the pinto beans, black beans, and corn. Mix well to combine. Even the top before sprinkling it with cheese. Cover the cooker with lid and continue to cook for 10-15 minutes more or until the cheese has melted.

5. Garnish with toppings of your choice and enjoy!

Serving: 6

Nutritional Facts: Calories - 519; Carbohydrates - 74g; Fats - 16g; Protein - 24g

Slow-Cooker Lamb with Olives and Potatoes

Ingredients

- 2.5 lbs. Lamb shanks, cut crosswise into (1.5 inches a piece)

- 1 1/4 lbs. Small potatoes, cut in halves

- tbsp. Almond Flour

- Large Shallots, cut into wedges (about half inch)

- tbsp. Lemon extract

- Cloves garlic, minced

- 1 tbsp. Grate lemon zest

- 3/4 cups Low-sodium chicken broth

- Sprigs of rosemary

- tbsp. Extra virgin olive oil

- 1/2 cup Dry white wine

- 1 cup of green olives, pitted and cut into halves

Directions

1   Add Garlic, shallots, potatoes, rosemary, and lemon zest in the slow cooker. Season with salt and pepper.

2   In a small mixing bowl, add a tablespoon of almond flour and broth. Mix and whisk before adding to the slow cooker.

3   Add the remaining 3 tablespoons of the almond flour on a plate.

4   Season lamb meat with salt and pepper and dip it in flour to coat. Shake to remove flour that didn't stick to the meat.

5   Preheat a large skillet and heat oil over medium-high heat. Cook meat in batches until all sides are brown before transferring to the slow cooker.

6   Add wine to the remaining meat juice on the skillet and cook, stirring to remove bits sticking to its bottom. Continue cooking until the liquid volume is reduced in half before adding to the slow cooker.

7   Cover slow cooker and set to cook for 7 hours on low or 3 ½ hours on high. After the allotted time, add olives, stir and continue cooking for 20 minutes more.

8   Once done, transfer dish to a platter. Serve with sauce taken from remaining cooking liquid and added with lemon juice

Serving: 4

Nutritional Facts (per serving): Calories - 521; Carbohydrates - 26.49g; Fats - 15.82; Protein – 69.32g

Slow-Cooked Lemon Asparagus

Ingredients

- 2 lbs. Asparagus

For the sauce:

- ½ cup Low-sodium chicken broth
- 1 lemon, sliced
- 2 cloves Garlic, minced
- 1 tsp. Basil
- 1 tsp. Garlic salt
- 4-6 tbsp. Lemon juice
- ¼ tsp. Red pepper flakes
- ½ tsp. Salt
- ½ tsp. Black pepper

Directions

1. Place the asparagus at the bottom of the cooker.

2. Mix all the sauce ingredients together in a small mixing bowl. Pour the mixture over the asparagus. Put lemon slices on top and cover the cook with lid.

3. Cook for about 2-4 hours on low (or 1-2 hours on high).

Serving: 8

Nutritional Facts: Calories — 31; Carbohydrates — 6.27g; Fats — 0.28g; Protein — 3g

Slow Cooker Mediterranean Eggplant

Ingredients

- 1 lb. Eggplant, peeled and chopped into 1-inch cubes
- 4 oz. Grass-fed feta cheese, crumbled
- 1 Large red bell pepper, seed removed and chopped
- 1 Large zucchini, chopped
- 4 Plum tomatoes, diced
- 1 Large onion, peeled and diced
- 4 cloves Garlic, peeled and minced
- 1 tbsp. Olive oil
- 2 tsp. Dried basil
- Salt
- Black pepper
- 4 pcs. Whole wheat pita bread (optional)

Directions

1. Pour the olive oil to the cooker.

2. Add the eggplant, zucchini, tomato, bell pepper, onion, basil, and garlic. Season with salt and pepper. Toss well so that the oil coats the ingredients.

3. Cover the cooker with the lid and cook on high for about 3 hours (or for about 5 hours on low).

4. Once done, add the feta cheese. Serve with pita bread if desired.

Serving: 4

Nutritional Facts (without the bread): Calories - 341; Carbohydrates - 50g; Fats - 11g; Protein - 13g

Slow Cooker Mushroom Bolognese

Ingredients

- 4 Cloves of garlic, minced

- 2 tbsp. Olive oil

- 1 Onion, finely chopped

- 2 tbsp. Tomato paste

- 1 Celery stalk

- 1 Carrot, finely chopped

- ½ tsp. Dried Rosemary

- 1/8 tsp. Ground nutmeg

- 1 tbsp. Balsamic vinegar

- 1/8 tsp. Red pepper (crushed)

- ½ tsp. Sugar

- ¼ cup Dry red wine

- 28-oz Crushed tomatoes in a can

- 1 pack of14-16 oz. White button mushrooms

Directions

1. Add white button mushrooms to the food processor and blend lightly to have it coarsely chopped but not pureed. Set aside for later use.

2. Preheat a large skillet on medium-high heat before adding olive oil. Sauté garlic, onions followed by carrots and celery. Add seasoning – salt and pepper to taste. Cook for about 3 minutes.

3. Add tomato paste, crushed pepper, nutmeg, and rosemary and continue to cook for 2 minutes. This will allow vegetables to soften and get a brownish color. Deglaze with the balsamic vinegar and wine. Stir using a wooden spoon to detach burn bits sticking to the bottom of the pan. Transfer the content into the slow cooker, stirring in tomatoes and sugar. Also, add the mushroom, stir, and cover with the lid. Cook on high for 4-6 hours. If you want longer cooking time, adjust to low setting and cook for 8-10 hours.

Serving: 4

Nutritional Facts (per serving): Calories -129; Carbohydrates - 14.3 Fats - 7.46g; Protein –3.14g

Slow Cooker Ratatouille

Ingredients

- 1 Large eggplant, chopped
- 4 Zucchini
- 1 cup Fresh basil, chopped
- 1 Orange bell pepper, chopped
- 1 cup Grape tomatoes, chopped
- 1 Large onion, chopped
- 6 cloves Garlic, minced
- 2 tbsp. Tomato paste
- 1 tsp. Dried oregano
- 2 tbsp. Coconut oil
- ½ -1 tsp. Sea salt
- 1 tsp. Ground pepper
- ¼ tsp. Crushed red pepper

Directions

1. Except for the basil, put all the ingredients into the slow cooker. Cover with the lid and cook on low for about 5-6 hours (or 3-4 hours on high). Once done, the veggies should be soft but not mushy. If the ratatouille is watery, just remove the lid and adjust to high in the last hour.

2. Before serving, mix in the basil. Serve this dish together with quinoa or brown rice.

Serving: 8

Nutritional Facts: Calories - 127; Carbohydrates - 23g; Fats - 5g; Protein - 5g

Slow Cooker Turkey Chili

Ingredients

- ¾ lb. Ground turkey meat
- 28-oz. can
- 3 Cloves garlic
- 2 tbsp. Olive oil
- 1 tbsp. Ground cumin
- 3 tbsp. chili powder
- ½ tsp. Cayenne pepper
- 3 tbsp. Tomato paste
- 1 Onion, chopped
- 1 tbsp. Dried oregano
- Kosher salt
- 28-oz. Fire-roasted canned tomatoes (diced)
- 2 2/3 cups Low-sodium chicken broth
- ¼ cup unsweetened cocoa powder
- 1 tbsp. Dried oregano
- 2 tbsp. Red wine vinegar
- 2 15-oz. Pinto beans in a can (strained and rinsed)
- 2 cups crushed corn tortilla chips
- 1 whole tortilla for serving

Directions

1. Heat a nonstick pan over medium-high heat and then pour olive oil. Add tomato paste along with chili powder, cayenne, and cumin. Stir until the mixture almost dries up and the oil is turning brick red in color.

2. Add the ground turkey meat seasoned with salt. Continue cooking until ingredients are well-blended before transferring the mixture to the slow cooker.

3. Add tomatoes, cocoa powder, oregano, vinegar, chicken broth, and 1 tsp. salt to the skillet and cook over medium-high heat for 2 minutes. Bring to simmer.

4. Add tomato mixture, crushed tortilla chips, onions, beans, and garlic and stir thoroughly. Secure the cover and continue cooking for 6-8 hours on low.

5. If the chili mixture needs thinning, you may add chicken broth. Serve with scallions and tortilla chips with grass-fed cheddar cheese.

Slow-Cooker Vegetable Curry with Tofu

Ingredients

- 1 x .16-oz Extra firm tofu, drained and pressed
- 1 Small eggplant, chopped
- 1 ½ cups bell pepper, sliced
- ¾ cup Peas
- 1 Medium onion, chopped
- 1 x 14.5-oz can Lite coconut milk
- 1 cup Vegetable broth
- ¼ cup Thai green (or red) curry paste
- 1 tbsp. Ginger, minced
- 1 tbsp. Coconut sugar
- ½ tsp. Turmeric
- 1 tsp. Salt
- Brown rice or quinoa, for serving (optional)

Directions

1. Put the vegetable broth, coconut milk, coconut sugar, curry paste, turmeric, ginger, and salt into the slow cooker. Whisk to combine well.

2. Add the eggplant, peppers, onions, and peas. Stir to combine and cover the cooker with lid. Cook on high for about 3-4 hours.

3. While the curry is cooking, chop the tofu to bite-size pieces. Put a large pan over medium heat. Pour olive oil and cook the tofu until golden. Set aside.

4. In the last 30 minutes of cooking time, add the tofu to the cooker. Once done, spoon over bowls of brown rice or quinoa if you want.

Serving: 4

Nutritional Facts (without the rice or quinoa): Calories - 425; Carbohydrates - 27g; Fats - 32.33g; Protein 16.53g

Thai Peanut Chicken Salad

Ingredients

For the salad:

- 4 x 6-oz. Chicken breasts

- 1 cup Peanuts, chopped

- 1 cup Purple cabbage, shredded

- 1 cup Red pepper, finely diced

- 1 cup Carrots, shredded

- ¼ cup Green onion, diced

- ½ cup Cilantro, chopped

For the sauce:

- 1 cup Nonfat Greek yogurt

- ½ cup Peanut butter, smooth

- ¼ cup Lime juice

- 1 tbsp. Soy sauce

- 2 tsp. Freshly ground ginger

- Salt

Directions

1. Put the chicken breast into the slow cooker, cover with the lid, and cook on high for about 1 ½ hours.

2. Meanwhile, combine all the salad ingredients into a large bowl, toss, and set aside.

3. Combine all ingredients for the sauce in a small bowl and stir well, to blend. Set aside.

4. Once the chicken breasts are done, shred them using two forks. Put into a container and let it cool. Mix in with the salad ingredients once cooled.

5. Pour the sauce over the salad and mix well to combine. Serve with a toast, over greens or on lettuce cups.

Serving: 6-8

Nutritional Facts: Calories - 256; Carbohydrates - 11g; Fats - 13g; Protein - 25g

Vegan Tofu Tikka Masala

Ingredients

- 1 16-oz Pack of Extra firm Tofu, drained and cubed
- cloves of garlic, minced
- 1 White onion, diced
- 1 Red bell pepper, chopped
- medium carrots, sliced
- 1 1/2 cups Potatoes, diced
- cups cauliflower florets
- 1 15-oz. can Tomato sauce
- 1 15-oz. can Coconut milk
- ½ tbsp. Pure maple syrup
- 1 tbsp. garam masala
- ½ tbsp. Freshly grated ginger
- 1 tsp. coriander
- ½ tsp. ground turmeric
- ¼ tsp. paprika
- Freshly ground black pepper
- ¾ cup frozen peas
- ¼ tsp. cayenne pepper
- 1 ½ teaspoons cumin
- ½ tsp. salt
- Fresh chopped cilantro, for garnishing

Directions

1   Combine garlic, garam masala, cayenne pepper, fresh ginger, paprika, diced onion, cauliflower florets, diced potatoes, sliced carrots, coconut milk, tomato sauce, maple syrup, fresh ginger, cumin, coriander, turmeric, cayenne pepper, salt and black pepper.

2   Stir to combine ingredients

3   Add in tofu cubes, and lightly stir before finally cooking on low for 6-7 hours or for 3-4 hours on high.

4   Before serving, stir in peas and cook without covering for 5-10minutes. Garnish with cilantro.

Serving:4-6

Nutritional Facts (per serving): Calories - 303; Carbohydrates -35.7 g; Fats- 11.5g; Protein - 14.8g

Snacks

Baked Sweet Potatoes in Slow Cooker

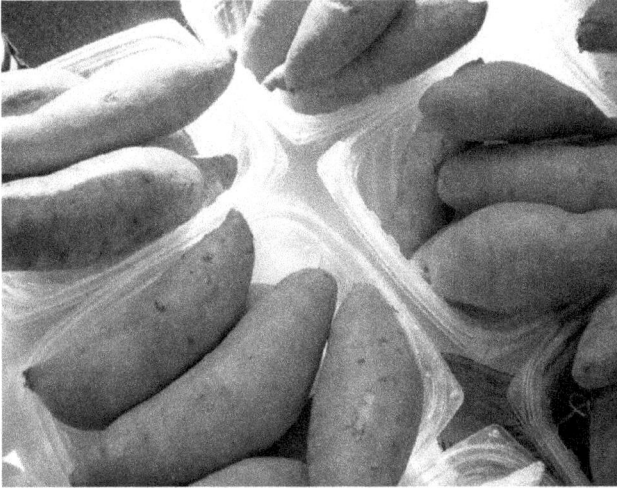

Ingredients

- 3 Large sweet potatoes, scrubbed

- 2 tsp. Olive oil

Directions

1. Rub oil on the potatoes and wrap each with foil. Put in the cooker and cover with lid. Cook on low for about 5-7 hours until fork-tender.

2. Remove from crockpot, remove the foil, and cut the potatoes into half lengthwise.

Serving: 6

Nutritional Facts (per half potato): Calories - 142; Carbohydrates - 32g; Fats - 0g; Protein - 4g

Cherry-Pistachio Brie

Ingredients

- ½ cup Dried cherries, snipped

- ½ cup Pistachios, toasted and coarsely chopped

- ¼ cup Cherry preserves

- 2 x 8-oz. rounds Grass-fed Brie cheese

- 1 tbsp. Cognac (or brandy)

- Pear slices, to serve

Directions

1. In a mixing bowl, mix the cherries, cherry preserves, cognac (or brandy).

2. Place one round of Brie at the bottom of the cooker, scoop half of the cherry mixture onto the top of the Brie. Add the second Brie on top of the cherry mixture and layer again with the remaining half of the cherry mixture.

3. Cover the cooker and cook on high for about 1- 1 ¼ hours (or for 3 hours on low) or until the cheese has softened but not yet melted.

4. Transfer to a serving platter and sprinkle with pistachios. Serve with pear slices on the side.

Serving: 20

Nutritional Facts: Calories - 166; Carbohydrates - 20g; Fats - 8g; Protein - 6g

Easy Slow-Cooked Cinnamon Pecans

Ingredients

- 3 cups Raw pecans, sliced
- 1 tbsp. Cinnamon
- ¼ cup Pure maple syrup
- 1 ½ tsp. Pure vanilla extract
- ¾ tsp. Salt
- 1 ½ tbsp. Coconut oil, optional

Directions

1. Lightly grease the crock with nonstick cooking spray.

2. Put all the ingredients except the pecans and mix. Add the pecans, cover the cooker, and put on low for about 2 hours.

3. After 2 hours, stir the nuts then cook again for another hour on low setting.

4. Once done, transfer the nuts to a cooking sheet and break up lumps. Set aside to cool. Enjoy!

Serving: 14 (serving size of 30g)

Nutritional Facts (per 30g): Calories- 181; Carbohydrates- 7g; Fats- 17.2g; Protein- 2.6g

Fruit Salsa

Ingredients

- 3 tbsp. Cornstarch

- 4 tsp. White vinegar

- 1 x 11 oz. can Mandarin oranges, undrained

- 1 x 8.5-oz. Sliced peaches, undrained

- ¾ cup Pineapple tidbits

- 1 Medium onion, chopped

- ½ Medium green pepper, chopped

- ½ Medium sweet red pepper, chopped

- ½ Medium yellow peppers, chopped

- 3 garlic cloves, minced

- 1 oz. Whole-wheat tortilla chips

Directions

1. Put the vinegar and cornstarch into the cooker and stir until smooth. Add the garlic, onion, pepper, and fruits.

2. Cover the cooker with lid and cook on high for about 2-3 hours or until a rich, thick consistency is achieved. Remember to stir from time-to-time. Serve with

3. Cover and cook on high for 2-3 hours or until thickened and heated through, stirring occasionally. Serve with whole-wheat tortilla chips.

Serving: 6

Nutritional Facts (¼ cup with tortillas): Calories — 102; Carbohydrates — 24g; Fats — 0.58g; Protein — 1.66g

Quinoa Energy Bars

Ingredients

- ⅓ cup Quinoa, uncooked
- ½ cup Raisins
- ⅓ cup Dried apples, roughly chopped
- ⅓ cup Roasted almonds, roughly chopped
- 2 tbsp. Almond butter
- 2 tbsp. Pure maple syrup
- 1 cup Unsweetened vanilla almond milk
- 2 Large eggs
- ½ tsp. Cinnamon
- 2 tbsp. Chia seeds
- Pinch of salt

Directions

1. Coat the crock with nonstick spray and line the bottom with parchment.

2. Put the maple syrup and almond butter in a microwave-safe bowl and microwave for about 30 seconds or until the butter is creamy. Remove from microwave and whisk.

3. Add the cinnamon, salt, and almond milk until everything is mixed well. Whisk in the eggs and add to the remaining ingredients. Mix well until everything is combined.

4. Pour the mixture into the pot and cook on low for about 3 ½- 4 hours or until the top of the quinoa mixture is already set.

5. Run a knife around the sides and remove the crock from the cooker. Refrigerate to cool thoroughly. Cut into bars and enjoy!

Serving: 8

Nutritional Facts (serving size of 71g): Calories - 174; Carbohydrates - 20.1g; Fats - 8.4g; Protein - 6.1g

Slow-Cooked Baked Oatmeal Bars

Ingredients

- 2 cups Rolled oats

- 1 cup Banana, mashed

- 2 eggs

- 1 ½ cups 1% Milk

- ½ tsp. Vanilla extract

- 1 tsp. Vanilla liquid stevia

- ½ cup Ground flaxseed

- 2 tsp. Ground cinnamon

- 1 tsp. Baking powder

- ½ tsp. Salt

For toppings (optional):

- Fresh blueberries

- Dried cherries

- Shredded unsweetened coconut

Directions

1. Using a stand mixer, blend the eggs, mashed banana, vanilla extract, vanilla liquid stevia, and milk.

2. In a separate mixing bowl, mix the remaining ingredients except for the toppings.

3. Add the dry ingredients into the wet and blend until they're well combined.

4. Line a parchment paper, extending to the sides of your crockpot.

5. Pour in the batter and spread evenly. Make sure that the top is evened out.

6. If you're using the toppings, sprinkle them on sections at the top and press them into the batter.

7. Secure the lid and cook under low heat for 8 hours.

8. Hold the ends of the parchment and transfer the oatmeal onto a cutting board. Divide into 16 bars. Serve or store in an airtight container.

Serving: 8

Nutritional Facts (per 1g bar): Calories - 168; Carbohydrates - 25.1g; Fats - 4.6g; Protein - 7.9g

Slow Cooker Mushrooms

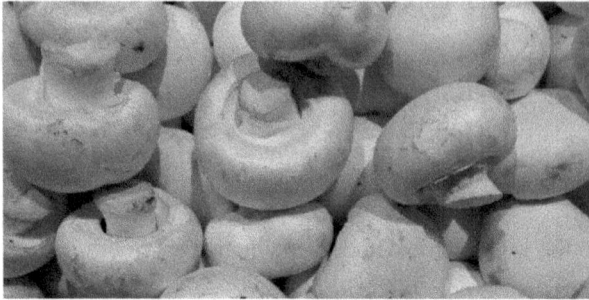

Ingredients

- 1 lb. White button mushrooms
- 4 cups Flat-leaf parsley, finely chopped
- 3 cloves Garlic, finely chopped
- 2 tbsp. Olive oil
- 1 tsp. Salt
- ¼ tsp. Ground black pepper

Directions

1. Trim off the ends of the mushrooms, leaving a little portion of the stem. Tidy them up with a damp towel.

2. Cut each mushroom into quarters then put them into the cooker together with the rest of the ingredients. Mix well to combine. Cook on high for about 2-3 hours.

3. Serve them with toothpicks.

Serving: 4

Nutritional Facts: Calories - 110; Carbohydrates - 8g; Fats - 7g; Protein - 5g

Slow Cooker Soy & Lime Chicken Wings

Ingredients

- 2 lb. Chicken wings
- ¼ cup Reduced-sodium soy sauce
- ¼ cup Balsamic vinegar
- 4 tsp. Cornstarch
- 3 tbsp. Honey
- 3 tbsp. Lime juice
- 2 cloves Garlic, minced
- 1 tsp. Sriracha sauce
- 1 tsp. Ginger powder
- 2 tsp. Sesame seeds
- 2 tbsp. Chives, chopped
- Zest of one lime

Directions

1. In a large mixing bowl, mix the lime juice, lime zest, Sriracha sauce, honey, soy sauce, vinegar, ginger powder, and garlic.

2. Put the chicken wings in the slow cooker. Pour the soy sauce mixture, covering every chicken wing. Stir to coat evenly.

3. Cover the cooker with lid and cook on high for about 3-4 hours (or on low for 6-7 hours).

4. In a small bowl, dissolve cornstarch in a tablespoon of water. Add it to the chicken, cover with lid, and cook for additional 10-12 minutes or until the sauce thickens.

5. Garnish with chives and sesame seeds before serving.

Serving: 4

Nutritional Facts: Calories- 384; Carbohydrates- 20.99g; Fats- 8.91g; Protein- 52.35g

Slow Cooker Quinoa Energy Bars

Ingredients

- ⅓ cup Quinoa, uncooked
- ½ cup Raisins
- ⅓ cup Dried apples, roughly chopped
- ⅓ cup Roasted almonds, roughly chopped
- 2 tbsp. Almond butter
- 2 tbsp. Pure maple syrup
- 1 cup Unsweetened vanilla almond milk
- 2 Large eggs
- ½ tsp. Cinnamon
- 2 tbsp. Chia seeds
- Pinch of salt

Directions

1. Coat the crock with nonstick spray and line the bottom with parchment.

2. Put the maple syrup and almond butter in a microwave-safe bowl and microwave for about 30 seconds or until the butter is creamy. Remove from microwave and whisk.

3. Add the cinnamon, salt, and almond milk until everything is mixed well. Whisk in the eggs and add to the remaining ingredients. Mix well until everything is combined.

4. Pour the mixture into the pot and cook on low for about 3 ½- 4 hours or until the top of the quinoa mixture is already set.

5. Run a knife around the sides and remove the crock from the cooker. Refrigerate to cool thoroughly. Cut into bars and enjoy!

Serving: 8

Nutritional Facts (serving size of 71g): Calories - 174; Carbohydrates - 20.1g; Fats - 8.4g; Protein - 6.1g

Tandoori Chicken Panini

Ingredients

- 1 ½ lb. Boneless, skinless chicken breasts
- ¼ cup Reduced-sodium chicken broth
- 2 cloves Garlic, minced
- 2 tsp. Fresh ginger, minced
- 1 tsp. Paprika
- ¼ tsp. Salt
- ¼- ½ tsp. Cayenne pepper
- ¼ tsp. Ground turmeric
- 6 Green onions, chopped
- 6 tbsp. Chutney
- 6 Whole-grain Naan flatbreads

Directions

1. Put the chicken breasts, ginger, garlic, paprika, turmeric, cayenne, salt, and broth into the cooker. Cover the cooker with lid and cook on low for about 3-4 hours or until the chicken is tender.

2. Once done, transfer the chicken to a plate and shred it using two forks. Return it to the cooker and add the green onions.

3. Spread chutney on one side of each flatbread then top with chicken mixture. Top again with flatbread, chutney side down.

4. Cook on an indoor grill or panini maker for about 6-8 minutes or until golden. Using a knife, cut the panini in half before serving.

Serving: 6

Nutritional Facts (per ½ panini): Calories - 351; Carbohydrates - 44g; Fats - 6g; Protein - 27g

Thai Curry Snack Mix

Ingredients

- ⅔ - 1 cup goji berries (or dried pineapple), chopped

- 5 cups Raw mixed nuts, some chopped and halved

- 1 cup Pumpkin seed

- ¼ cup Coconut sugar

- 2 tbsp. Tamari sauce (or coconut aminos)

- ½ tbsp. Red curry powder

- ½ tsp. Thai red chili powder

- 2 tsp. Paprika

- 1 tsp. Onion powder

- 1 tsp. Garlic

- 1 tbsp. Red pepper flakes

- 2 tbsp. Coconut oil

- 1 tsp. Sea salt

- ½ tsp. Black pepper

Directions

1. Lightly grease the crock of your cooker and put the all the ingredients except for the dried goji berries or pineapple. Mix everything until well combined.

2. Cook on medium for 2 hours, stirring once every 30 minutes (or on high for 1- 1 ½ hours, stirring once halfway), monitoring the progress of the candy. While cooking, line a baking sheet with parchment.

3. Once done, lay out the candied nuts on the baking sheet to cool.

4. Add the dried goji or pineapple and serve. You can also store it in a ziplock or sealed container for up to 2 weeks.

Serving: 8 (serving size of ⅓ cup)

Nutritional Facts: Calories - 230; Carbohydrates - 11.5g; Fats - 17.5g; Protein - 6.

Turmeric Tortillas

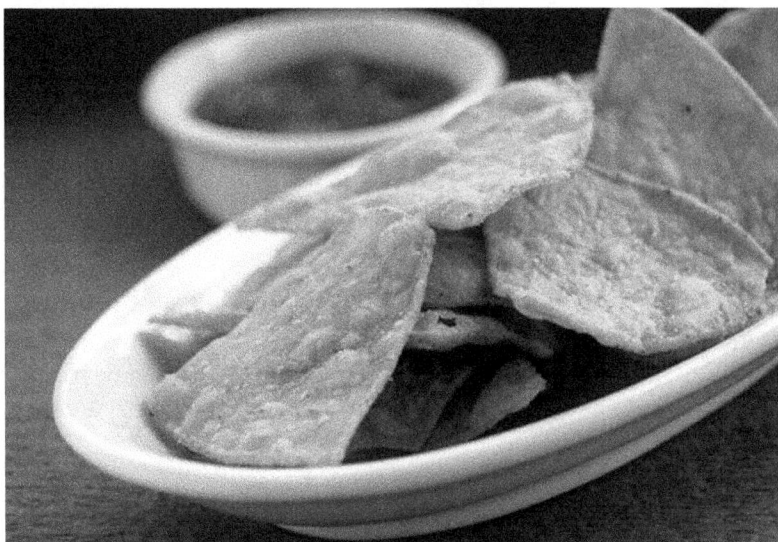

Ingredients

- 1 cup of cassava flour

- ½ tsp. Coconut flour

- ½ tsp. Baking powder

- ½ tsp. Turmeric powder

- 2/3 cups Warm water

- ½ tsp. Apple cider vinegar

- ½ tsp. Fine sea salt

- 3 tbsp. Extra virgin olive oil

Directions

1. In a large mixing bowl, combine coconut flour, cassava flour, sea salt, baking powder, and turmeric powder.

2. In another mixing bowl, add warm water, apple cider vinegar, and extra virgin olive oil. Mix to blend.

3. Combine the liquid mixture to the dry mixture and blend thoroughly using a spatula. Use your hands in kneading to form a smooth dough.

4. Divide the smooth dough into two halves. Further, divide each half into three equal portions to give you 6 dough balls in all. Using a rolling pin, roll each ball between two sheets of parchment papers to form a thin circular sheet of dough about 6 inches in diameter.

5. While stacking the rolled-out pieces of tortillas, leaving a sheet of parchment paper in-between layers to prevent them from sticking together.

6. Preheat a nonstick skillet in a stove over medium-high heat. Cook tortilla for about 2 minutes each, uncovered until bubbles appear on the surface and edges becomes brown. Flip to cook the other side for 1 ½ - 2 minutes more

7. Serve warm or store in the fridge or freezer for later use.

Serving: 4

Nutritional Facts (per serving): Calories - 83; Carbohydrates - 13.49g; Fats - 3.11; Protein – 0.52g

Soup

Anti-Inflammatory Veggie Soup

Ingredients

- A cup of coconut milk
- 1 tsp. Turmeric
- 1 tsp. Ginger, freshly grated
- 2 lbs. Carrots, chopped
- Salt and pepper to taste
- 6 cups of bone broth

Directions

1. Combine all ingredients in slow cooker and cook on low heat for 10 hours. Blend in the cooker using an immersion blender for a smooth and creamy soup. Serve hot or warm.

Serving: 4

Nutritional Facts (per serving): Calories - 560; Carbohydrates - 23.22g; Fats - 32.75; Protein – 42.23g

Bone Broth

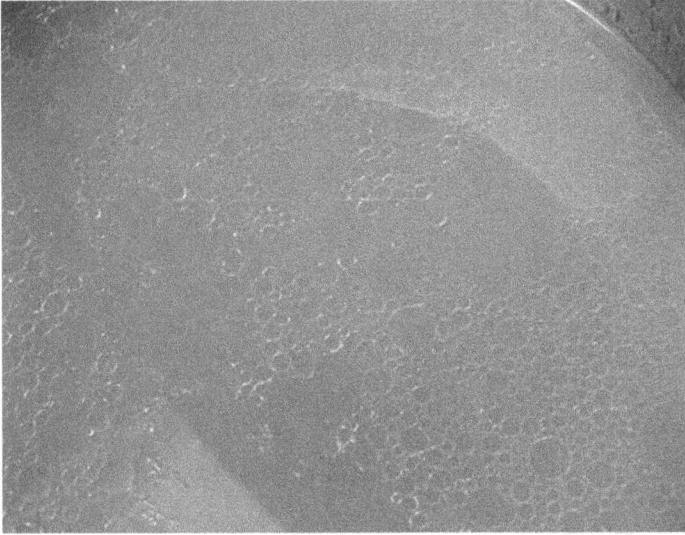

Ingredients

- 1 Whole Fish or 1 whole chicken
- 1 tbsp. Peppercorns (alternative: a dash of paprika)
- 2 Sweet bay leaves
- Vegetable scraps (carrots, celery, onions, etc.)
- A cup of water

Directions

1. Add everything in the slow cooker and cook on low setting for 24 hours. When bones easily crumble when pressed lightly, have it ready to serve.

Serving: 6

Nutritional Facts (per serving): Calories - 189; Carbohydrates - 12.86; Fats - 7.65; Protein – 16.47

Broccoli, Turmeric and Ginger Soup

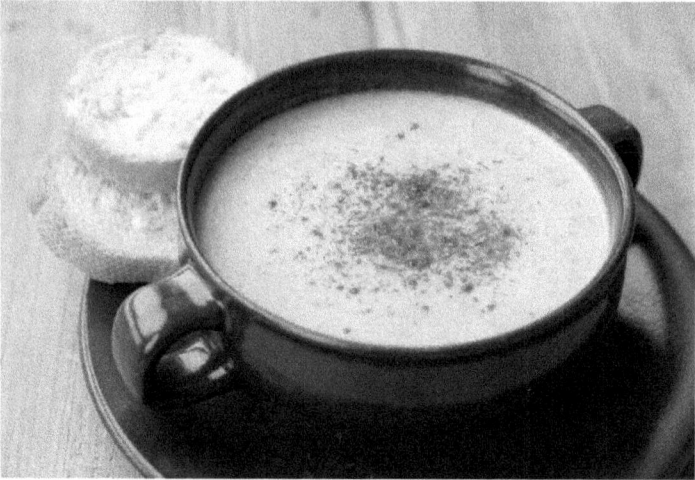

Ingredients

- 8 cups Broccoli florets

- 2 tbsp. Ginger, chopped

- 4 cups Leeks, chopped

- 6 cups Stock

- 2 tbsp. Butter

- 1 tsp. Ground turmeric

- 1 tbsp. Sesame oil

- A pinch of black pepper

- 1 tsp. Salt

Directions

1. Start by melting the butter in a large pan over medium heat. Cook the leeks for about 8 minutes, stirring occasionally until they're cooked through.

2. Put the broccoli, ginger, turmeric, stock, and salt into the slow cooker. Transfer the leeks as well. Cover with lid and put the setting on low. Cook for 3-4 hours or until the broccoli is tender.

3. Using an immersion blender or food processor, process the broccoli mixture until smooth and creamy.

4. Transfer to serving bowls. Serve with yogurt and whole-wheat bread on the side.

Serving: 8

Nutritional Facts: Calories - 126; Carbohydrates - 11g; Fats - 7g; Protein - 7g

Butternut Squash Soup

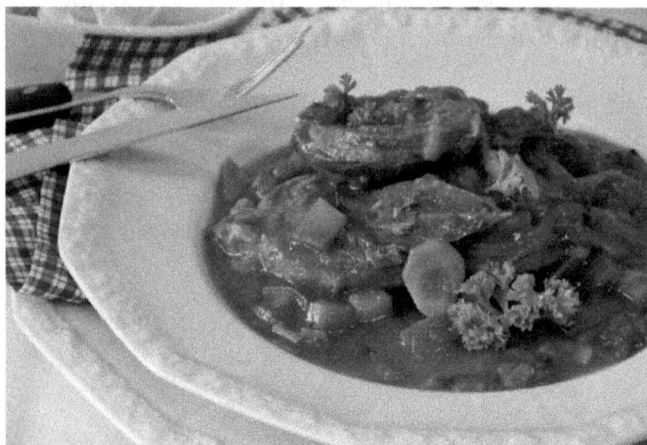

Ingredients

- 1 medium (about 8 cups) butternut squash, peeled, seeded and diced
- 1 Carrot, peeled and roughly chopped
- 1 White onion, peeled and roughly chopped
- 1 apple, cored and roughly chopped
- ½ cup Unsweetened coconut milk
- 2 cups Vegetable stock
- 4 cloves Garlic, peeled and minced
- 1 sprig Fresh sage
- ⅛ tsp. Cayenne
- Pinch of ground cinnamon and nutmeg
- ½ tsp. Salt
- ¼ tsp. Black pepper, freshly ground

Directions

1. Put the butternut squash, carrot, apple, onion, garlic, sage, cinnamon, nutmeg, cayenne, and vegetable stock in the crock of slow cooker. Season with salt and black pepper. Toss well to combine. Cook for about 3-4 hours on high (or 6-8 hours on low) or until the squash is tender and can be easily mashed using a fork.

2. Discard the sage and add the coconut milk.

3. With the use of an immersion blender, puree the soup until smooth. Alternatively, use a regular blender to puree the soup. Work in batches if needed.

4. Stir in the cayenne. Season with additional salt and pepper if desired. Serve warm.

Serving: 8

Nutritional Facts (per cup): Calories - 129; Carbohydrates - 25g; Fats - 3.8g; Protein - 2.7g

Cauliflower Bolognese With Zucchini Noodles

Ingredients

For the Bolognese:

- tsp. of dried oregano flakes
- 1 head of cauliflower (cut into florets)
- 1 tsp. Dried basil flakes
- Garlic cloves, minced
- ¾ cups Red onion, diced
- ½ cup Vegetable broth, low-sodium
- ¼ tsp. Red pepper flakes
- 14-oz. cans Diced tomatoes (no salt added)
- Salt and pepper to taste

For the Pasta

- 4 Zucchinis (spiraled using blade A)

Directions

1 Add all Bolognese ingredients into the slow cooker and cook on high for about 3-5 hours.

2 Once done, crush cauliflower using a potato masher or fork to break up florets and have your Bolognese

3 Spoon over Bolognese on bowls of zucchini noodles.

Serving: 6

Nutritional Facts (per serving): Calories - 35; Carbohydrates - 7.54 Fats - 0.37; Protein –7.54

Slow-Cooker Black Bean Soup

Ingredients:

- 1 Large Onion, chopped
- Red bell peppers, cored and chopped
- Carrots, chopped
- Cloves garlic, minced
- Jalapeno peppers, diced
- cups Low-sodium Vegetable stock
- 15-oz. cans of black beans, rinsed and drained
- 1 Bay leaf
- tsp. Ground cumin
- 2 tsp. Chili powder
- 2 tsp. Kosher salt
- 1/2 tsp. Cayenne pepper
- Optional toppings:
- Chopped fresh cilantro
- Diced avocados

Directions

1   Throw in all ingredients in the slow cooker and stir to combine. Cook on low setting for 6-8 hours or 3-4 hours when set on high. Once done and all vegetables are cooked and tender but not mushy, remove the bay leaf.

2   Serve with desired garnish or toppings.

Serving: 8

Nutritional Facts (per serving): Calories - 257; Carbohydrates - 39.03 Fats - 5.63; Protein −15.19

Slow Cooker Kale and Quinoa Soup

Ingredients

- 3 cups Kale, chopped

- ½ cup Dry quinoa

- 2 Medium potatoes, peeled and diced

- 2 cups Cannellini beans (canned), drained

- 4 cups Low-sodium vegetable broth

- 1 Medium onion, diced

- 2 twigs Fresh rosemary

- ¼ tsp. Black pepper, freshly ground

- 2 tbsp. Extra-virgin olive oil (plus more to drizzle)

Directions

1. Make cream by adding 1 cup of beans in a bowl and blending it using an immersion blender. You can also use a traditional blender or food processor.

2. Put the cream together with the broth, remaining cup of beans, potatoes, onions, rosemary, oil, and black pepper into the cooker. Cook for 2-4 hours on high (or 4-6 hours on low). Add the kale and quinoa in the last 30 minutes of cooking.

3. Drizzle with olive oil before serving.

Serving: 6 (serving size of 1 ½ cups)

Nutritional Facts: Calories - 360; Carbohydrates - 56g; Fats - 11g; Protein - 11g

Healing Slow-Cooked Lamb & Thyme Soup

Ingredients

For the lamb stock:

- 1 lamb shank

- 2 carrots, sliced

- 4 cups water

- 1 onion, quartered

- 2 bay leaves

- Coconut oil (to drizzle)

- Salt

- Black pepper

For the soup:

- 2 Sweet Potatoes, chopped into small pieces

- 2 Small potatoes, chopped into small pieces

- 2 Carrots, chopped into small pieces

- 2 Tomatoes, chopped into small pieces

- 1 Onion, finely chopped

- 2 cloves Garlic

- ½ cup Red wine

- 1 tsp. Fresh oregano

- 1 tsp. Turmeric, finely grated

- 1 tsp. Fresh thyme

- ½ tsp. Cumin

- Salt

- Black pepper

- Parsley, for garnish

Directions

1. To make the stock, rub some salt and pepper on the shank.

2. Place a skillet on medium-high heat, some oil, and sear the meat on both sides. Once done, place the shank on the slow cooker along with the stock ingredients and cook on low for about 9-10 hours.

3. When the cooking time is up, remove the shank and transfer to a chopping board. Chop the shank into small pieces and set aside.

4. Transfer the stock into a container, letting it cool completely refrigerating it. Once cooled, you can find some fat on the surface. Skim them off and put the stock back to the slow cooker.

5. Put the vegetables into the cooker along with the red wine, onion, garlic, thyme, turmeric, oregano, cumin, salt, and pepper. Cook for 6-8 hours under low setting. Add the lamb shank to the soup 1 hour before the end of cooking time. Sprinkle with parsley before serving.

Serving: 6

Nutritional Facts: Calories - 345; Carbohydrates - 31.09g; Fats - 8.42g; Protein - 37.33g

Healthy Chicken Chili

Ingredients

- 2 lbs. boneless skinless chicken breasts
- 1 x 15oz. can Pinto or kidney beans, rinsed and drained
- 1 x 15oz. can Black beans, rinsed and drained
- 1 x 14.5 oz. can Fire-roasted tomatoes (diced), undrained
- 1 x 4 oz. can Green chilies (chopped), undrained
- 2 cups Low-sodium chicken broth
- 1 Medium jalapeño pepper, finely chopped
- 1 Medium green bell pepper, chopped
- 1 Medium onion, chopped
- 1 tbsp. Chili powder
- 1 ½ tsp. Ground cumin
- 1 tsp. Paprika
- ½ tsp. Kosher salt
- ¼ tsp. Cayenne
- Salt
- Black pepper, freshly ground

For the toppings (optional):

- Fresh cilantro (or green onions), chopped
- Avocado, diced (or guacamole)
- Plain, nonfat Greek yogurt
- Pickled jalapeños

Directions

1. Place the onions and peppers (bell pepper and jalapeños) at the bottom of the crock.

2. In a small bowl, incorporate the paprika, chili powder, cumin, cayenne, and salt. Mix well to combine. Using half of the spice mixture, season the chicken.

3. Place the chicken atop the peppers and onions. Add the chilies, tomatoes, and 1 cup of broth plus the rest of the seasoning.

4. Set the cooker on low for 6-7 hours (or on high for 3-4 hours).

5. Once the chicken is tender, transfer the chicken to a cutting board then put the beans to the cooker. If the sauce is too thick, adjust by adding more broth until you achieve desired consistency.

6. Meanwhile, cut the chicken to bite-size pieces or you can shred it using two forks. Return the chicken to the cooker and mix to combine well. Season with salt and black pepper. Serve with toppings of choice.

Serving: 6

Nutritional Facts: Calories - 422; Carbohydrates - 41g; Fats - 11g; Protein - 59g

Mexican Chicken Soup

Ingredients

- 1 tsp. Chili powder
- 3 Whole chicken breasts (boneless and skinless)
- 1 tsp. Ground cumin
- Freshly ground black pepper
- 28-oz. can whole or diced tomatoes, with juice
- 15-oz. can black beans, drained and rinsed
- 3 cups low-sodium chicken broth
- 10-oz. can diced tomatoes with green chilies
- 1 Onion, chopped
- 4-oz. Tomato paste
- 1 Red bell pepper, chopped
- 1 Yellow bell pepper, chopped
- 1/2 lime (extract juice)
- 1 can Chipotle pepper in adobo
- Kosher salt

Directions

1. Place chicken meat in the slow cooker. Season it with chili powder, cumin, salt and pepper to taste. Also, add tomatoes, tomatoes with chilies, tomato paste, chipotle pepper, red and yellow peppers, black beans, and chicken broth. Mix and cover the slow cooker. Cook for 8 hours on low or you may set it for 5 hours on high heat.

2. When done, pour lime juice over dish and stir. Transfer chicken

meat to a plate and use forks to shred it into fine pieces. Return shredded pieces to the slow cooker and adjust taste by adding some seasonings if needed.

3. Serve hot in a bowl with avocado and turmeric tortillas with cilantro leaves as garnish.

Serving: 8

Nutritional Facts (per serving): Calories - 186; Carbohydrates - 26.62 Fats - 3.23; Protein –14.81

Parsnip – Split Pea Soup

Ingredients

- 1 tbsp. Olive oil
- 1 Onion, diced
- Cloves of garlic, minced
- 2 large parsnips, chopped
- 2 large carrots, chopped
- 1 lb. Dried green split peas
- 1 tsp. Dried thyme
- 1 tsp. Poultry seasoning (optional)
- 2 Bay leaves
- cups water
- Mineral salt
- Pepper

Directions

1. Preheat a nonstick skillet and sauté onion, garlic, carrots and parsnips using olive oil for about 4 minutes.

2. Add sautéed veggies to the slow cooker along with the rest of the ingredients.

3. Cook for about 8 hours on low.

4. When done, remove bay leaves and blend using an immersion blender. Blend well until desired consistency is achieved. See to it that the mixture is creamy and less chunky. Add seasoning according to desired taste.

Serving: 8

Nutritional Facts (per serving): Calories - 165; Carbohydrates - 29.37 Fats - 2.81; Protein –7.47

Roasted Red Pepper Tomato & Turmeric Soup

Ingredients

- 1 x 12-oz. Roasted red peppers
- 1 x 28-oz. can Crushed tomatoes
- 2- 3 cups vegetable broth
- 1 White onion, diced
- 4 cloves Garlic, minced
- 1 tbsp. Powdered turmeric
- 1 tbsp. Coconut oil
- ½ tsp. Dried basil
- ½ tsp. Dried thyme
- ½ tsp. Pepper

Directions

1. Place skillet over medium-high heat and pour oil. Sauté the garlic and onion for about 2-3 minutes until soft and fragrant. Blend in spices and cook for another 30 seconds.

2. Transfer the sautéed spices to the cooker. Add the tomatoes, peppers, and broth. Cover the cooker with lid and cook on low for 6-7 hours (or for 3-4 hours on high).

3. Once done, let it cool for a bit. Transfer contents (you may work in batches) to a blender and process. If you have an immersion blender, you can use it instead of the traditional blender. You may need some broth to adjust to your desired consistency.

Serving: 4

Nutritional Facts: Calories - 117; Carbohydrates - 20.08g; Fats - 4.2g; Protein - 3.21g

Slow-Cooked Chicken Noodle Soup

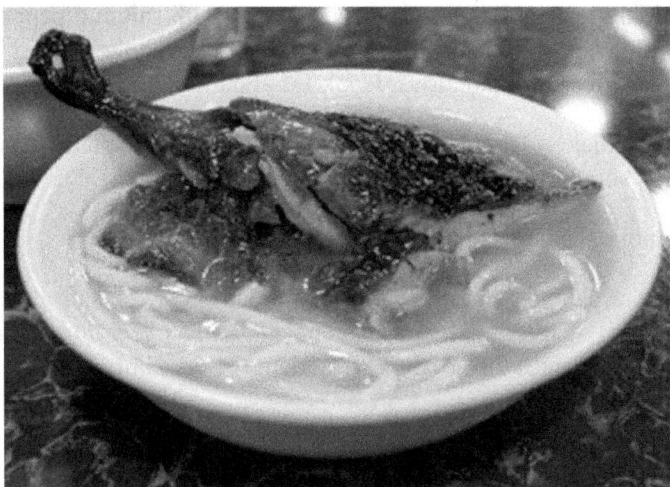

Ingredients

- 8 oz. Egg noodles
- 1 ½ lb. Boneless, skinless chicken breasts
- 10 cups Low-sodium chicken broth
- 3 Carrots, peeled and sliced into coins
- 1 large Onion, chopped
- 3 cloves Garlic, minced
- 2 stalks Celery, sliced
- 4 tsp. Fresh thyme sprigs
- 4 tsp. Fresh rosemary sprigs
- 1 Bay leaf
- Kosher salt
- Freshly ground black pepper

Directions

1. Combine the chicken, carrots, celery, onion, garlic, rosemary, thyme, and bay leaf in the slow cooker. Season with salt and pepper before pouring the broth into the slow cooker. Cover the cooker with lid and put the setting on low. Cook for about 6-8 hours.

2. Take chicken from the cooker and transfer on a plate. Using two forks shred the chicken breasts.

3. Remove the herbs and bay leaf, then discard.

4. Put the chicken shreds back into the slow cooker and also add the noodles. Cover with lid and cook again on low for about 20-30 minutes or until the noodles are al dente. Serve hot.

Serving: 8

Nutritional Facts: Calories - 240; Carbohydrates - 13.1g; Fats- 7g; Protein - 28.9g

Slow Cooker Savory Superfood Soup

Ingredients

- 2 cups Kale, coarsely chopped
- 2 cups Carrots, sliced
- 1 Large sweet potato, cut into ½-inch cubes
- 1 cup Fresh green beans
- 2 x 15 oz. cans Black beans, drained and rinsed
- 2 cups Organic vegetable juice
- 2 cups Low-sodium vegetable broth
- ½ cup Fresh cilantro, chopped
- 1 Small onion, diced
- 1 Clove garlic, minced
- 1 tsp. Chili powder
- 1 tsp. Cumin
- ½ tsp. Red pepper flakes, crushed
- ½ tsp. Black pepper
- Kosher or sea salt

Directions

1. Put all the ingredients together in the cooker, cover with lid, and cook on low for 6-8 hours or until the vegetables are tender. Put the kale in the last 5 minutes of cooking.

Serving: 8

Nutritional Facts (per serving): Calories -157; Carbohydrates - 32g; Fats - 1g; Protein - 7g

Slow Cooker Winter Vegetable Medley

Ingredients

- 2 ½ cups Butternut or acorn squash, peeled and chopped
- 2 ½ cups Baby carrots
- 2 ½ cups Vegetable Broth
- 1 Onion, sliced
- 1 tsp. Thyme
- ½ tsp. Sea salt
- Chives or parsley, chopped (to garnish)

Directions

1. Put everything into the cooker, close with lid, and cook on low for about 4-6 hour or until the veggies are fork-tender. Garnish with chives or parsley before serving.

Serving: 4

Nutritional Facts (per serving): Calories - 128; Carbohydrates - 28g; Fats - 1g; Protein - 4g

Spicy Fajita Soup

Ingredients

- 1/2 cup Corn, thawed

- 2 tbsp. Chili powder

- 2 green peppers, julienned

- 2 medium yellow onions, sliced

- 1 Chipotle pepper in adobo sauce, chopped

- 1 tbsp. Garlic, minced and chopped

- 4 cups of chicken broth

- 2 cups olive oil

- 12 Whole wheat tortillas, divided into 8

- 2 scallions, sliced

- 1 14-oz. can of diced tomatoes

- 1 cup Grass-fed or organic Monterey Jack cheese

- 2 scallions, sliced

Directions

1. Add onions, garlic, corn, tomatoes, peppers, chipotle, broth and a tablespoon of chili powder into the slow cooker. Season with salt and pepper and set to cook for 4-6 hours.

2. Preheat the broiler

3. Preheat a deep skillet in a stove over medium heat and add the olive oil. Fry tortilla pieces for about 1-2 minutes or until brown. Drain in a paper towel and season with salt and the remaining chili powder.

4.   Preheat the broiler. Ladle cooked soup into oven-proof bowls with 2 tablespoons of grass-fed cheese on top and place each bowl in a sheet pan.

5.   Place sheet pan with bowls of soup in the broiler and cook for about 1-2 minutes or until cheese is brown and bubbly. Serve.

Serving: 8

Nutritional Facts (per serving): Calories - 432; Carbohydrates - 56.37 Fats - 95.45; Protein –49.67

Strawberry Beet Soup

Ingredients

- 6 cups Fresh strawberries, hulled

- 2 lb. Beets, peeled

- 4 cups Bone broth or chicken broth

- 1 cup Buttermilk

- ¼ tsp. Freshly ground black pepper

- ½ tsp. Salt

- ¼ cup Hemp seeds (or ¼ cup sesame seeds)

Directions

1. In a slow cooker, put the beets, salt, pepper, and broth. Cover the cooker with lid and put the setting on high. Cook for about 2 to 2 ½ hours or until the beets are tender.

2. Using an immersion blender (or food processor) puree the beet mixture until smooth.

3. Add the strawberries and process again until smooth.

4. Divide into bowls. Garnish each bowl with 2 tbsp. buttermilk and half tablespoon hemp seeds. Serve while hot.

Serving: 8

Nutritional Facts: Calories- 227; Carbohydrates- 24g; Fats- 5g; Protein- 12g

Vegan Slow-Cooker Detox Coconut Soup

For the Broth:

- cans of 13.5-oz Coconut milk

- cups Vegetable broth

- stalks Lemongrass, smashed

- pcs Fresh ginger (2 inches in length a piece), peeled and sliced

- 2 garlic cloves, minced

- 1 scallion

- Kosher salt

- Juice extract of 2 limes

For Toppings:

- 5-oz Baby spinach

- cups Sliced snow peas

- Scallions, julienned

- ½ cup Unsweetened coconut flakes

- Basil leaves

- 1 cup Bean sprouts

- Mint leaves

- Cilantro leaves

- Red Fresno chili, julienned

- Lime wedges, for serving

Directions

For the Broth:

1. Combine lemongrass, garlic, ginger, scallions, and coconut milk with the vegetable broth in the slow cooker. Set on low and cook for 7 hours until you can smell the broth's aroma.

2. Remove the lemongrass stalks, garlic cloves, ginger, and scallions from the broth. Enhance the flavor by adding lime juice. Season with salt to taste.

3. Also, add in snow peas and spinach and allow it to sit for 7-10 minutes. Stir before serving.

4. Serve in bowls topped with bean sprouts, scallions, coconut flakes, cilantro, mint, basil, and chili. With more lime while still hot.

Servings: 8

Nutrition Facts: Calories - 115; Carbohydrates - 18g; Fat - 31g; Protein - 3g

Seafood

Healthy Slow-Cooked Salmon

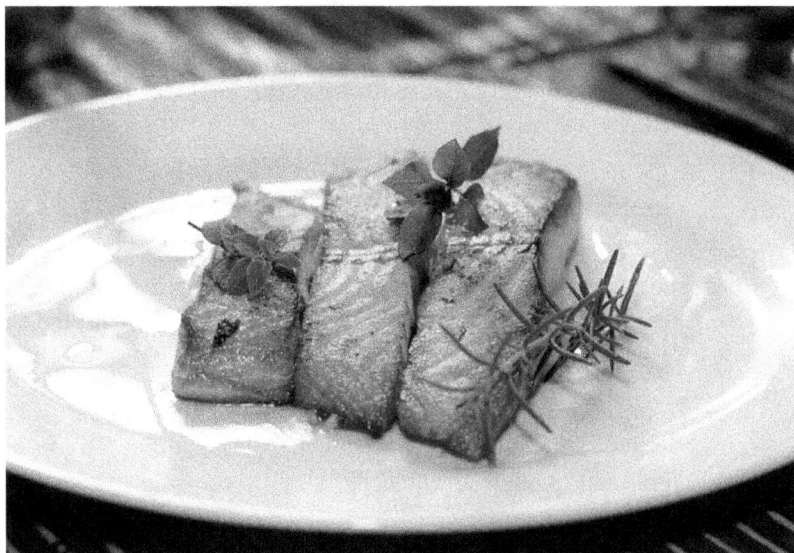

Ingredients

- 2 lb. Salmon fillets with skin-on

- 1 ½ cup Vegetable Broth

- 1 Onion, sliced

- Salt

- Black pepper, freshly ground

- Lemon juice from 1 lemon

- 1 lemon, sliced into rounds

Directions

1. Cut the salmon into individual servings. Rub some salt and pepper on each side then sprinkle with lemon.

2. Line the bottom of the crock with a square foil or parchment. The excess edges will make it easier for you to lift the fish from the cooker later on.

3. Place the sliced onion and lemon in a single layer at the bottom of the crock. Put the salmon fillets over them with the skin-side down. If the salmon doesn't fit in a single layer only, put another parchment or foil over the first layer of salmon and lay the rest (still with the skin-side down).

4. Pour the broth over salmon. If you manage to have a single layer of salmon only, add enough broth to cover the fish fillets. If you have two layers, add enough to come partway up the side of the second layer.

5. Secure the lid cover and cook on low heat for about 1-2 hours. Check the salmon after an hour and continue checking every 20 minutes after that. The salmon should be done at 145°F in the thickest part of the fish.

6. Transfer the salmon by carefully lifting the sides of the foil or parchment, draining the liquid in the process. Serve immediately.

Serving: 6

Nutritional Facts (per serving): Calories - 391; Carbohydrates - 9.2g; Fats - 23g; Protein - 34.9g

Hearty Slow-Cooked Catfish Stew

Ingredients

- 1 ½ lb. Catfish fillets, cut into 2-inch pieces
- 1 x 14.5-oz. can Whole tomatoes
- 4 oz. Mushrooms, sliced
- ¼ cup Dry white wine
- 1 Green bell pepper, cut into 1-inch piece
- 2 small zucchini squash, sliced
- 1 Large clove garlic, minced
- 1 Large onion, sliced
- ½ tsp. Dried leaf basil
- ½ tsp. Dried leaf oregano
- 2 tbsp. Extra-virgin olive oil
- 1 tsp. Salt
- ⅛ tsp. Black pepper
- Parsley, for garnish

Directions

1. Start by placing all the ingredients into a 5-quart slow cooker. Mix everything well to combine.

2. Cover the cooker with lid and switch setting on high for about the about 3 ½ - 5 ½ hours. Garnish with parsley before serving.

Serving: 6

Nutritional Facts: Calories - 225; Carbohydrates - 17g; Fats - 8g; Protein- 21g

Lemony Salmon & Dill

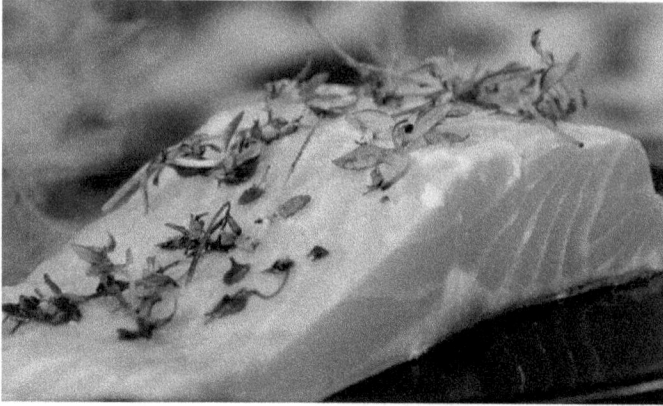

Ingredients

- 2 lb. Salmon fillet
- 1 lemon, sliced
- 2 Garlic cloves, minced
- 1 tsp. extra-virgin olive oil
- A handful of fresh dill
- Salt
- Pepper

Directions

1. Generously coat the crock with nonstick cooking spray or line the bottom with parchment.

2. Rub the fish with olive oil then season it with dill, garlic, salt, and pepper. Put it into the cooker. Top with lemon slices and cook on low for about 2 hours (or on high for about an hour).

Serving: 2

Nutritional Facts (per serving): Calories - 346; Carbohydrates - 9.4g; Fats - 12.9g; Protein - 51.2g

Scalloped Potatoes with Salmon

Ingredients

- 1 x 16-oz. Salmon, drained and flaked
- 4 - 5 potatoes, sliced
- 10.75-oz. Cream of mushroom soup (alternative: cream of celery soup)
- ½ cup Onion, chopped
- ¼ cup Water
- 3 tbsp. Flour
- Dash nutmeg
- Salt
- Black pepper

Directions

1. Grease the crock of the slow cooker with nonstick spray.

2. Layer half of the potatoes at the bottom, sprinkle with 1 ½ tbsp. of flour, and lightly sprinkle with salt and pepper. Spread half of the salmon flakes on top and sprinkle with ¼ cup of onion. Repeat these to make another layer.

3. In a bowl, combine the soup and water. Pour into the cooker. Add the nutmeg.

4. Cover the cooker with lid and cook on low for about 7-9 hours or until the potatoes are fork-tender.

Serving: 6

Nutritional Facts: Calories - 438; Carbohydrates - 24g; Fats - 28g; Protein - 22g

Slow Cooker BBQ Shrimp

Ingredients

- 2 lbs. Shrimp, peeled, deveined

- 1 cup Organic barbecue sauce

- 3 tbsp. Grass-fed butter

- 3 tbsp. Worcestershire sauce

- 2 tsp. Garlic, minced

- Salt

- Black pepper

- Lemon wedges, for garnish

Directions

1. Put all the ingredients (except for lime wedges) into the cooker and mix well. Cook on low for an hour.

2. Serve with lime wedges and vegetables on the side.

Serving: 4

Nutritional Facts (per serving): Calories - 408; Carbohydrates - 33.12g; Fats - 10.29g; Protein - 46.43g

Slow Cooker Red Curry With Cod

Ingredients

- 1 lb. Codfish fillet
- 340g Carrots, julienned
- 2 x 15-oz. can Light coconut milk
- 1 Red bell pepper, sliced
- 3 tbsp. Red curry paste
- 1 tbsp. Curry powder
- 1 tsp. Ground ginger
- 1 tsp. Garlic powder
- Salt
- Black pepper
- 1 cup brown rice, cooked
- Green onion, chopped (for garnish)

Directions

1. Stir in the coconut milk, curry powder, ground ginger, garlic powder, and curry paste into the slow cooker. Add the carrots and bell peppers then carefully add the cod fillet into the sauce.

2. Cover the cooker with lid and cook on low for about 2 hours.

3. Once done, slice the cod to bite-size pieces. Season the sauce with salt and pepper. Add the cod back to the sauce, stir well, and ladle to serving bowls with brown rice. Garnish with chopped green onions and enjoy!

Serving: 4

Nutritional Facts (per serving): Calories - 611; Carbohydrates - 30.8g; Fats - 46.79g; Protein - 24.69g

Slow Cooker Fisherman's Stew (Cioppino)

Ingredients

- 1 x 28-oz. can Crushed tomatoes with juice
- 1 x 8-oz. can Tomato sauce
- 1 cup Dry white wine
- ½ cup Onion, chopped
- ⅓ cup Olive oil
- ½ cup Parsley, chopped
- 2 tsp. Basil
- 1 tsp. Thyme
- 1 tsp. Oregano
- ½ tsp. Paprika
- ½ tsp. Cayenne pepper
- 3 cloves Garlic, minced
- 1 Green pepper, chopped
- 1 Hot pepper, chopped (optional)
- Salt
- Black pepper

For the seafood:

- 1 Seabass or other white fish fillets, deboned and cubed
- 1 doz. Clams (you can also use canned)
- 1 doz. Scallops
- 1 doz. Prawns
- 1 doz. Mussels

Directions

1. Put all ingredients (except for the seafood) into the slow cooker. Cover it with lid and cook on low for 6-8 hours.

2. In the last 30 minutes of cooking, add the seafood. Switch to high and stir occasionally. If you want a thinner liquid consistency, add ½ cup of water or broth.

Serving: 6

Nutritional Facts (per serving): Calories - 434; Carbohydrates - 27g; Fats - 16g; Protein - 39g

Slow Cooker Fish & Tomatoes

Ingredients

- 1 lb. Cod
- 1 x 15-oz. can Tomatoes, diced
- ¼ cup Low-sodium broth
- 1 Bell pepper, sliced
- 1 Medium onion, sliced
- 3 cloves Garlic, minced
- 1 tbsp. Rosemary
- ¼ tsp. Red pepper flakes
- ¼ tsp. Salt
- ¼ tsp. Black pepper

Directions

1. Place all the ingredients (except for the fish) into the slow cooker and mix well.

2. Season the fish with salt and pepper (or your preferred seasoning). Add it on top of the tomato mixture and cover the cooker with lid. Cook on low for 1-3 hours (or on high for 30 minutes to 1 ½ hours).

3. Divide into 4 portions and serve.

Serving: 4

Nutritional Facts: Calories - 130; Carbohydrates - 9g; Fats - 1g; Protein - 22g

Slow Cooker Garlic Shrimp Recipe

Ingredients

For the Creole seasoning:

- 2 tsp. Black pepper, freshly ground

- 1 tsp. Cayenne pepper

- 1 tbsp. Garlic powder

- 1 tsp. Onion powder

- 1 tsp. Dried leaf thyme

- 1 tsp. Dried leaf oregano

- 1 tbsp. Salt

- 1 tbsp. Paprika

- For the garlic shrimp:

- 1.5 lb. Extra-large (or jumbo) shrimp, peeled and deveined

- 1 tsp. Creole seasoning (see below)

- 4 tbsp. Grass-fed butter

- ¼ cup Olive oil

- 5 cloves Garlic, peeled and thinly sliced

- ⅛ tsp. Ground cayenne pepper

- ¼ tsp. Black pepper, freshly ground

- 1-2 tbsp. fresh parsley, minced (for garnish)

Directions

1. Prepare the creole seasoning by mixing all the creole seasoning together in a small mixing bowl. Get the required amount for the garlic shrimp recipe and store the remaining amount in a container. Keep in cool, dark storage.

2. For the garlic shrimp, put the butter, garlic, creole seasoning, oil, cayenne, and black pepper into the cooker. Cover and set on high for about 25-30 minutes.

3. Meanwhile, rinse the shrimp using cold water then pat them dry.

4. Add the shrimp into the butter mixture and stir well to coat. Cook on high for about 20-30 minutes, stirring halfway through cooking time. Once done, the shrimp should be opaque and pink.

5. Transfer to a serving dish and garnish with parsley.

Serving: 4-6

Nutritional Facts (per serving): Calories - 307; Carbohydrates - 9g; Fats - 18g; Protein - 28g

Slow Cooker Soy-Ginger Steamed Pompano

Ingredients

- 1 Whole pompano, cleaned, scaled and gutted
- 1 bunch Leeks
- ¼ cup Chinese cooking wine
- ¼ cup Tamari sauce
- ¼ cup Sesame oil
- 1 x 2-inch Ginger, cut into thin strips
- 2 tbsp. Honey
- For garnish:
- 6 cloves Garlic, minced and fried
- 1 bunch Cilantro, roughly chopped

Directions

1. Create diagonal slits on both sides of the fish.

2. In a mixing bowl, incorporate the cooking wine, soy sauce, honey, ginger, and sesame oil.

3. Layer the leeks at the bottom of the slow cooker. Place the fish on top and pour the sauce on top of it.

4. Switch the cooker on high and cook for 1 hour.

5. Once done, transfer the fish together with its sauce to a serving dish. Top with cilantro and fried garlic. Serve and enjoy!

Serving: 4

Nutritional Facts (per serving): Calories - 465; Carbohydrates - 14.8g; Fats - 30g; Protein - 34g

Slow-Cooked Lemon Caper Halibut

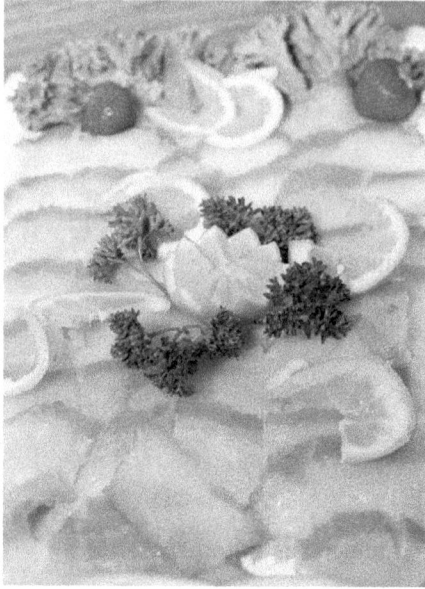

Ingredients

- 4 Halibut Fillets

- 2 Lemons

- ½ cup Chicken broth

- 1 tbsp. Dried basil

- 1 tsp. Garlic, minced

- 1 tbsp. Capers

- 2 tbsp. Grass-fed butter

- Salt

- Black pepper

Directions

1. Slice one of the lemons into 10 thin rounds and arrange at the bottom of the cooker. Set aside remaining lemon, cut in wedges. Layer halibut on top of the lemon slices and pour the broth. Season with dried basil, salt, and pepper.

2. Set on low and cook for 2-3 hours or until the internal temperature in the thickest part of the halibut is 145°F.

3. Heat the butter in a small saucepan and add the capers. Cook until the butter starts to brown.

4. Transfer the halibut to a serving plate and drizzle with the caper sauce. Garnish with lemon wedges.

Serving: 6

Nutritional Facts (per serving): Calories - 291; Carbohydrates - 6g; Fats - 11.7g; Protein - 41g

Slow Cooker Miso-Poached Salmon

Ingredients

- 2 pcs. Salmon Fillet

- 1 cup Mushrooms

- ½ cup Miso paste

- ½ cup Scallions, thinly sliced

- 3 cups Fish stock

- 1 x 2-inch piece Ginger, thinly sliced

- 2 tsp. Salt (or fish sauce)

Directions

1. Mix the miso paste, scallions, ginger, and stock in the cooker. Cook on low for about 4 hours.

2. After 4 hours, switch to high. Place the salmon fillets and mushrooms into the cooker and cook for another 10 minutes. Season with fish sauce or salt before serving.

Serving: 2

Nutritional Facts: Calories - 393; Carbohydrates - 22g; Fats - 13.4g; Protein - 47g

Slow Cooker Pineapple-Ginger Poached Milkfish

Ingredients

- 500g Milkfish

- 1 Cup Pineapple chunks

- 1 Cup Pineapple juice

- ¼ cup White vinegar

- 1 x 2- inch piece Ginger, peeled and thinly sliced

- 4-5 Pieces Jalapeno Peppers

- 6 cloves Garlic, minced

- ½ tbsp. Black Peppercorns

Directions

1. Rub the milkfish with salt. Put everything, including the fish, into the cooker and cover the cooker with lid.

2. Cook on low for about 4 hours.

Serving: 4

Nutritional Facts (per serving): Calories - 260; Carbohydrates - 18.59g; Fats - 8.63g; Protein - 26.69g

Slow Cooker Seafood Medley

Ingredients

- 1 lb. Shrimp, peeled and deveined
- 1 lb. Bay scallop
- 1 lb. Crabmeat
- 2 x 10.75-oz. Cans cream of celery soup
- 21 ½ oz. 1% Milk
- 2 tbsp. Grass-fed butter
- 1 tsp. Old Bay Seasoning
- ¼ tsp. Salt
- ¼ tsp. Black pepper

Directions

1. Layer the scallops, shrimp, and crab at the bottom of the crock.

2. In a bowl, mix the milk and celery soup before pouring over the seafood. Add the spices and butter on top and cover the cooker with lid.

3. Cook on low for 3-4 hours. Serve over brown rice if desired.

Serving: 10

Nutritional Facts (per serving): Calories - 232.7; Carbohydrates - 8.9g; Fats - 8.8g; Protein - 28.1g

Slow Cooker Shrimp Creole

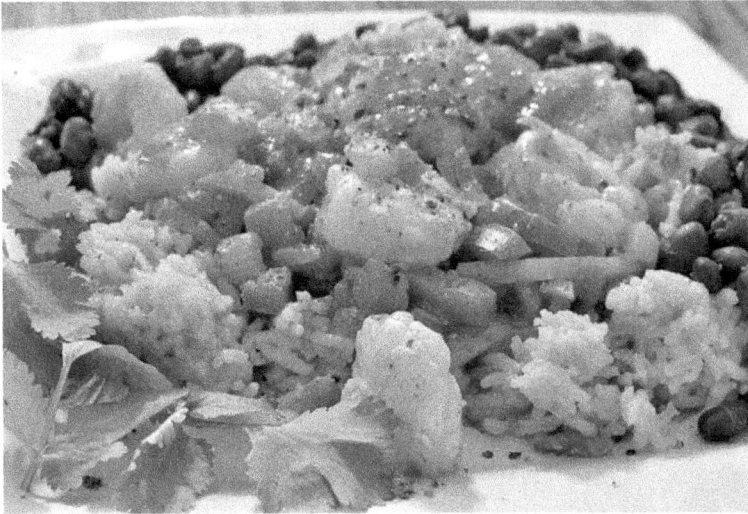

Ingredients

- 1 - 1.5 lb. Shrimp, deveined and shelled

- 1 x 28-oz. can Whole tomatoes, broken up

- 1 x 8-oz. can Tomato sauce

- 1 ½ cups celery, diced

- 1 ¼ cups onion, chopped

- 1 cup bell pepper, chopped

- 1 clove garlic, minced

- ½ tsp. Creole seasoning

- 6 drops Tabasco

- 1 tsp. Salt

- ¼ tsp. Black pepper, freshly ground

425

Directions

1. Place all the ingredients (except for the shrimp) into the cooker and cover the cooker with lid. Set on low and cook for about 6-8 hours. When using high heat, cook for 3-4 hours.

2. Add the shrimp in the last 30 minutes of cooking. Serve over cooked brown rice.

Serving: 2-3

Nutritional Facts (per serving): Calories - 388; Carbohydrates - 42g; Fats - 3g; Protein - 52g

Slow-Cooked Shrimp Scampi

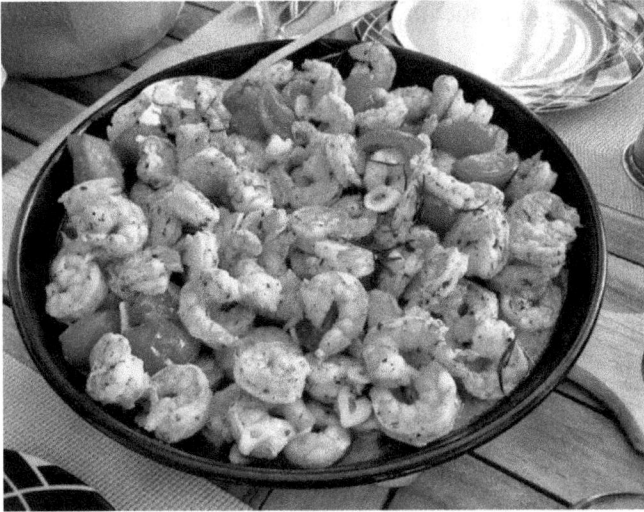

Ingredients

- 1 lb. Shrimp, peeled and deveined

- ½ cup White cooking wine

- ¼ cup Chicken bone broth

- 2 tbsp. Olive oil

- 2 tbsp. Grass-fed butter

- 2 tbsp. Parsley finely, chopped

- 1 tbsp. Garlic, minced

- 1 tbsp. Lemon juice

- ½ tsp. Red pepper flakes

- Salt

- Black pepper

Directions

1. Mix butter, red pepper flakes, lemon juice, garlic, olive oil, broth, wine, salt, and pepper in the cooker. Add the shrimp and cover.

2. Cook on low for about 2 ½ hours (or on high for 1 ½ hours). Once done, transfer to a serving dish and enjoy.

Serving: 4

Nutritional Facts (per serving): Calories - 256; Carbohydrates - 2.1g; Fats - 14.7g; Protein - 23.3g

Slow Cooker Seafood Stew

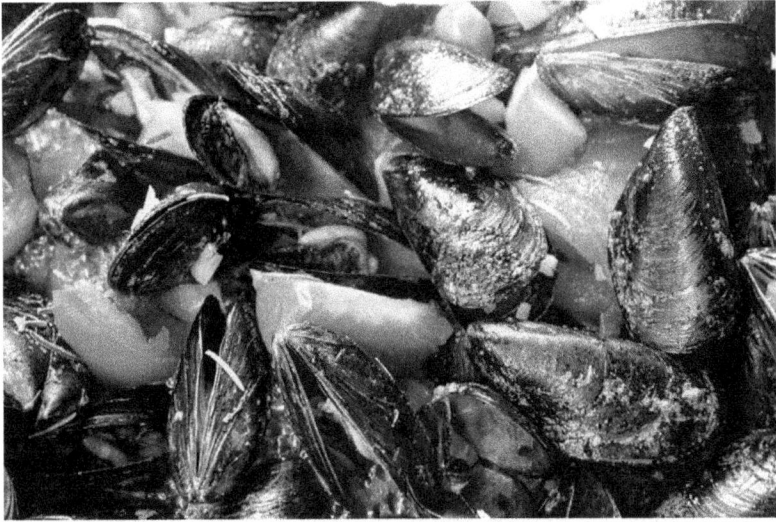

Ingredients

- 2 lb. Seafood (scallops, crab legs, large shrimp)

- 1 lb. Dutch baby potatoes, cut into bite-size pieces

- 1 x 28-oz. Crushed tomatoes

- 4 cups Vegetable broth

- ½ cup White wine

- ½ cup Medium onion, diced

- 3 cloves Garlic, minced

- 1 tsp. Dried basil

- 1 tsp. Dried thyme

- 1 tsp. Dried cilantro

- ½ tsp. Celery salt

- ¼ tsp. Red pepper flakes

- Pinch cayenne pepper

- ½ tsp. Salt

- ½ tsp. Black pepper

Directions

1. Put all ingredients (except for the seafood) into the slow cooker. Cover the cooker with lid and cook on low for 4-6 hours (or on high for 2-3 hours).

2. Add the seafood into the cooker, switch to high and cook for 30 minutes to 1 hour or until the seafood is completely cooked.

3. Ladle to bowls and serve with whole wheat bread if desired.

Serving: 6

Nutritional Facts (per serving): Calories - 236; Carbohydrates - 31g; Fats- 1g; Protein - 22g

Slow Cooker Spanish Sardines

Ingredients

- 2 lb. Pilchard Fish heads, cleansed
- 1 cup Olive oil
- 1 cup fish (or vegetable) stock
- 1 Carrot peeled, (round thin cuts)
- 1 bulb Garlic (cut into 2-inch cubes)
- 1 Dill pickle (sliced into small rounds)
- 1 Pickled jalapeño (sliced into small rounds
- 5 chilies
- 3 Bay Leaves
- 1 tbsp. Whole black peppercorn
- Salt

Directions

1. First, soak the fish in brine for about half an hour. Rinse and drain.
2. Arrange the carrots, pickles
3. Leave the fish in a brine solution for 30 minutes. Wash and drain.
4. Arrange in layers ingredients starting with carrots, garlic, pickles, jalapeno, chilies, bay leaves, garlic, and black peppercorns.
5. Arrange fish on top.
6. Add in olive oil and stock.
7. Sprinkle fish with a generous amount of salt.
8. Cook on low for 8 hours.

Serving: 8-10

Nutritional Facts (per serving): Calories - 383; Carbohydrates - 2.54g; Fats - 34.6g; Protein - 15.8g

Slow Cooker Spanish Shrimp and Quinoa

Ingredients

- 1 cup Quinoa, rinsed
- 1 x 10-oz. package Shrimp peeled, deveined, tail off
- 1 x 14-oz. can Fire-roasted tomatoes, drained
- 2 cups Vegetable Broth
- 1 cup Spinach
- ½ tsp. Cayenne pepper
- ½ tsp. Smoked paprika
- 1 tsp. Onion powder
- 1 tsp. Dried coriander
- 2 tbsp. Honey
- 1 tbsp. Worcestershire sauce
- 1 tbsp. Olive oil
- 1 tbsp. Lime juice
- Salt
- Black pepper

For garnish:

- 1 cup Green onion, chopped
- Grass-fed crumbled goat cheese
- Parsley and other herbs

Directions

1. Coat the crock with nonstick cooking spray.

2. Put the quinoa, shrimp, tomatoes, honey, Worcestershire sauce, spinach, onion powder, cayenne, coriander, paprika, lime juice, olive oil, and broth into the crock of the slow cooker. Mix well to combine.

3. Cover the cooker with lid and cook on low for about 3 - 3 ½ hours (or on high for 2 - 2 ½ hours).

4. Season with salt and pepper, give a good stir and transfer to bowls. Garnish crumbled goat cheese, green onions, parsley, and/or other herbs.

Serving: 4

Nutritional Facts (per serving): Calories - 345; Carbohydrates - 47g; Fats - 7g; Protein - 23g

Slow Cooker Tilapia

Ingredients

- 2 lb. Tilapia fillets, divided into 8 pieces
- 1 cup Mayonnaise
- Lemon juice from 1 lemon
- 1 tbsp. Fresh garlic

Directions

1. In a small mixing bowl, combine the mayonnaise, garlic, and lemon juice.

2. Brush the fillets with the mayonnaise mixture on both sides.

3. Line the bottom of the crock with aluminum foil. Make sure to have excess sides to serve as a handle. Layer the fish fillets on top.

4. Secure with cover and set cooking on low heat for about 3-4 hours.

Serving: 8

Nutritional Facts (per serving): Calories - 176; Carbohydrates - 5.25g; Fats - 7.32g; Protein - 22.94g

Slow-Cooked White Beans and Tuna

Ingredients

- 3 cans x 12 oz. White tuna in water drained and flaked
- 1 lb. Small white beans, soaked overnight drained
- 2 cups Tomatoes, chopped
- 6 cups Water
- 1 clove Garlic, crushed
- 2 sprigs Basil, finely chopped
- 4 tbsp. Olive oil
- Salt
- Black pepper, freshly ground

Directions

1. Pre-heat a large skillet over medium heat and add olive oil in. Sauté the garlic for 1 minute. Discard the garlic but retain the oil.

2. Add the beans into the slow cooker and pour the garlic-flavored oil over them. Pour the water, cover the cooker, and cook on high for about an hour.

3. After an hour, switch to low and cook for 4-7 hours more or until the beans are tender. (Note: The cooking time depends on the age of beans and your cooker. Just to make sure, monitor them after 4 or 5 hours.)

4. Switch the cooker off and then add the tuna, tomatoes, and basil. Season with salt and pepper. Serve and enjoy!

Serving: 6

Nutritional Facts: Calories - 472; Carbohydrates - 57g; Fats - 13g; Protein - 34g

Tuna Potato Casserole in Slow Cooker

Ingredients

- 4 potatoes, peeled and sliced

- 2 x 170g cans Tuna, drained

- 1 x 10.75-oz. can Cream of celery soup

- 2 cups Green peas

- 1 tbsp. Curry powder

- ¼ cup Water

Directions

1. Layer half of the tomatoes at the bottom of the cooker. Next, layer half of the veggies, tuna, and ½ tbsp. of curry powder. Repeat the layers.

2. Spoon the soup on top before adding the water.

3. Cover the cooker with lid and cook on low for about 7-10 hours or until the potatoes are fork tender.

Serving: 4
Nutritional Facts (per serving): Calories - 403.7; Carbohydrates - 53.8g; Fats - 8.2g; Protein - 29.2

Slow Cooker Moqueca with Tilapia & Shrimp

Ingredients

- 2 lb. Whitefish fillet, cut into bite-size pieces
- 1 lb. Shrimp, peeled and deveined
- 1 White onion, thinly sliced
- 1 Yellow bell pepper, thinly sliced
- 1 cup Tomatoes, diced
- 1 tbsp. Garlic, minced
- Lime juice from 1 lime
- 2 cups Coconut milk
- Salt
- Black pepper
- 1 bunch Cilantro, chopped (for garnish)

Directions

1. Assemble the tomatoes, bell peppers, onions, and garlic at the bottom of the cooker.

2. Add the lime juice and coconut milk. Set the cooker on high and cook for about an hour. Season with salt and pepper.

3. Layer the fish and shrimp above the mixture and switch the setting on high. Cook for another 20 minutes. Before serving, top the moqueca with cilantro.

Serving: 8

Nutritional Facts (per serving): Calories - 278; Carbohydrates - 5g; Fats - 15g; Protein - 32g

Meat and Poultry

Almond Butter Beef Stew

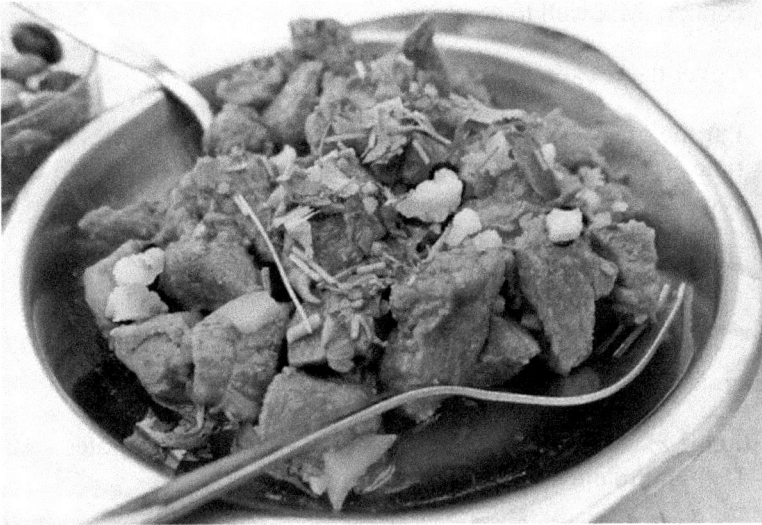

Ingredients

- 2 lbs. Round steak, cut into 1 ½-inch pieces
- 5 cups Bone broth or stock
- ½ cup Creamy, unsweetened almond butter
- 1 ½ cups Tomatoes, diced
- 2 cups Sweet potatoes, diced
- 1 cup Carrots, diced
- 1 ½ cup Green beans, roughly chopped
- 1 Large onion, finely chopped
- 2 Bay leaves
- 1 tbsp. Coconut oil
- 1 ½ tsp. Salt
- ¼ tsp. Black pepper

439

Directions

1. Except for the green beans, put all the ingredients into the slow cooker. Mix well to combine.

2. Cover the cooker with lid and cook on low for about 6-8 hours.

3. Put the green beans to the cooker in the last 30 minutes of cooking time, stirring again to mix everything. Cover with lid and continue cooking.

4. Before serving, remove the bay leaves. Enjoy!

Serving: 6

Nutritional Facts (per serving): Calories - 428; Carbohydrates - 10.79g; Fats - 18.44g; Protein - 52.22g

Balsamic Chicken and Mushroom Stroganoff

Ingredients

- 4 Boneless, skinless chicken breast fillets, cubed

- 1 cup 2% Plain Greek yogurt

- 1 x 16 oz. package Mushrooms, sliced

- 1 cup Chicken broth, fat-free

- 1 Yellow onion, diced

- 2 cloves Garlic, minced

- ½ tsp. Black pepper

- ½ tsp. Kosher or sea salt

Directions

1. Spread the chicken at the bottom of the cooker. Add in the garlic, onion, mushrooms, vinegar, and broth. Season with salt and pepper. Cover the cooker and set on high for 3-4 hours (or 5-6 hours on low).

2. Once done, stir in the yogurt. Serve with whole wheat pasta or brown rice if desired.

Serving: 8

Nutritional Facts (per serving): Calories - 187; Carbohydrates - 9g; Fats - 4g; Protein - 27g

Beef, Barley and Vegetable Stew

Ingredients

- Garlic cloves, minced
- 3 tbsp. Olive oil
- cups Chicken or beef broth, divided
- 1 lb. Beef chuck, divide and cut into 3
- ½ lb. of small potatoes, halved
- 1/2 cup Pearl barley
- Thyme sprigs
- 1 lb. Medium butternut squash, diced
- Salt and pepper to taste

Directions

1   Heal a tablespoon of olive oil on a large skillet over medium-high heat.

2   Season beef with salt and pepper and cook in the hot skillet until brown on all sides. Once done, transfer meat to slow cooker.

3   Add remaining oil and sauté garlic before adding thyme. When browned and you can smell the aroma, add 2 cups of broth. Continue cooking and stirring, scraping the bottom of the skillet to remove pieces sticking to its bottom.

4   Pour mixture into the slow cooker and add squash, potatoes, barley along with two remaining cups of water and 2 cups of broth. Secure cover and cook on high for 4 hours on high or 8 hours on low. Check afterward for tenderness. Once done, shred into pieces using forks. Check for desired taste and make the adjustment on the seasoning if needed.

Serving: 8

Nutritional Facts (per serving): Calories - 298; Carbohydrates - 32.02 Fats - 11.41; Protein –18.96

Chicken Meatballs in Slow Cooker

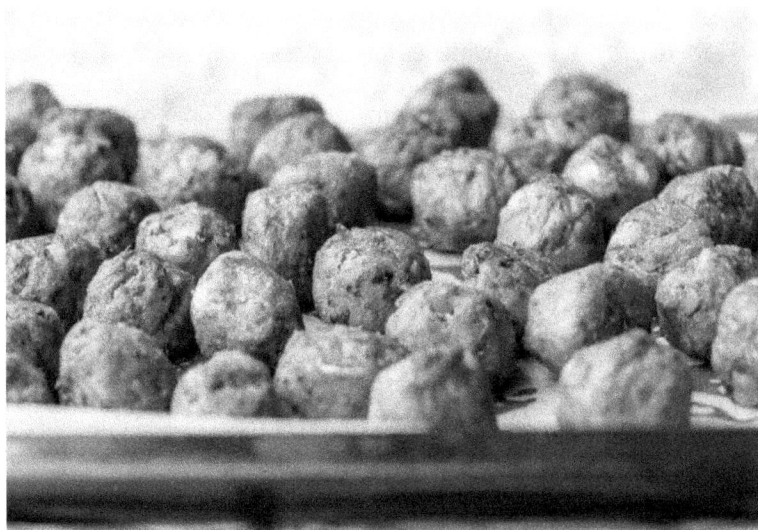

Ingredients

For the meatballs:

- 1 lb. Ground pork

- 2 tsp. Poultry seasoning

- 2 tsp. Dried parsley or cilantro

- 2 tbsp. Olive oil

- For the sauce:

- 1 cup Chicken broth

- 13.5 oz. Coconut milk

- 2 tbsp. Curry powder

- 1 tsp. Garlic powder

- ½ tsp. Salt

443

Others:

- ½ cup Heavy cream

- ½ Medium yellow or white onion, chopped

- 1 Large sweet potato, peeled and cubed

- 2 tbsp. Butter

Directions

1. Incorporate all meatball ingredients in a large mixing ball.

2. Make Ping-Pong sized meatballs and line them in a single layer at the bottom of the crock.

3. Into another bowl, combine all sauce ingredients and pour over the meatballs.

4. Top with onions, cubed potatoes, and butter.

5. Cover the cooker with lid and cook on high for about 4 hours (or 6-8 hrs. on low). Ensure that the meatballs are cooked through.

6. Stir in heavy cream and mix well before serving. Serve with rice if desired.

Serving: 4

Nutritional Facts: Calories - 623; Carbohydrates - 15g; Fats - 54g; Protein - 24g

Chicken Tomatillo Verde

Ingredients

- 4 x 6oz. Boneless, skinless chicken breasts
- 4 Tomatillos, husked and rinsed
- 2 x 15oz. cans Chickpeas drained and rinsed
- 1 cup packed Fresh basil leaves
- 2 cups Baby kale, chopped
- ½ Onion, minced
- ½ tsp. Salt
- ½ cup Sour cream (optional)

Directions

1. Put the tomatillos in the slow cooker, add 2 tbsp. water, and cover the cooker with lid. Set the cooker on high and cook for an hour or until the tomatillos are soft.

2. Once cooked, transfer the tomatillos on a plate and let cool for about 5 minutes.

3. Meanwhile, process the basil, kale, onions, and salt in food processor until finely chopped. Add the cooled tomatillos (depending on the processor you use, you may need to cut the tomatillos first) and process again until the consistency of salsa is achieved.

4. Put the chickpeas on the slow cooker (it's okay not to wash the cooker after the tomatillos) and place the chicken breasts atop the chickpeas. Drizzle with half amount of the salsa, cover with lid, and cook on low for about 1-2 hours or until the chicken is thoroughly cooked.

5. Divide the chicken between four plates and spoon the veggies (sauce and all) on top. Serve with the remaining salsa and sour cream (if desired).

Serving: 4

Nutritional Facts (with sour cream): Calories - 475; Carbohydrates - 26g; Fats - 14g; Protein - 66g

Cranberry Pork Roast

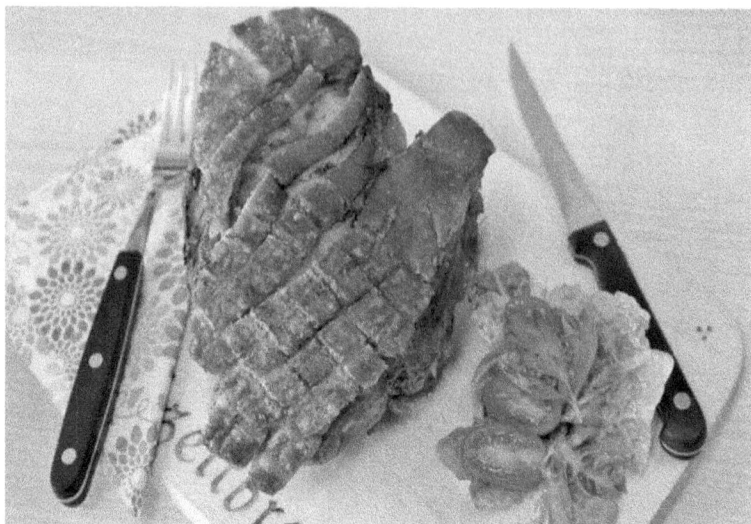

Ingredients

- 1 x 15oz. can Whole berry cranberry sauce

- lb. Bone-in pork shoulder

- ¼ cup Dried minced onion

- ¼ cup Honey

Directions

1. Put all the ingredients into the cooker and set on low for about 6-8 hours. Once done, shred the pork with a fork and serve with vegetables.

Serving: 8

Nutritional Facts (per serving): Calories - 298; Carbohydrates - 32.02 Fats - 11.41; Protein – 18.96

Cuban Beef

Ingredients

- 4 cups Cauliflower rice

- 2 lb. Beef chuck roast

- 1 x 6oz. can tomato paste

- 1 cup Beef broth

- ½ cup Cilantro, chopped

- 1 Poblano pepper, chopped

- 1 Medium white onion

- 2 tbsp. Olive oil

- 2 tbsp. Cumin

- 1 tbsp. Garlic

- 1 tbsp. Oregano

- 1 tbsp. Smoked paprika

- 1 Lime, cut into wedges

Directions

1. Cut the onion in half. Cut the first half into thin slices while the other half should be chopped.

2. Place a large pan over medium-high heat and pour olive oil. Once hot, sear the beef for 2 minutes on both sides.

3. Transfer the beef with oil and juices to the slow cooker. Add the sliced onions and poblano pepper. Pour in the broth then add the tomato paste, garlic, paprika, and cumin. Cover the cooker with lid and cook on low for 6-8 hours.

4. When the beef is already fork-tender, transfer it to a plate and shred

using forks. Once done, bring the shredded beef to the cooker and cook for another 30 minutes.

5. Serve over cauliflower rice with cilantro, chopped onions, and a lime wedge as toppings.

Serving: 4

Nutritional Facts : Calories- 615; Carbohydrates- 21.28g; Fats- 29.14g; Protein- 72.06g

Cuban Pork Tacos with Fried Plantains

Ingredients

For the marinade:

- ½ cup Orange juice
- ¼ cup Cilantro, chopped
- 3 cloves Garlic, peeled
- 2 tbsp. Olive oil
- ½ tsp. Red pepper or cayenne
- ½ tsp. Cumin
- ¼ tsp. Dried oregano
- 3 tbsp. Lime juice

In the crockpot:

- 1 lb. Lean pork or pork loin
- 1 Small white onion, chopped
- ½ tap. Salt
- ½ tsp. Black pepper

For toppings:

- 1 plantain, sliced and peeled
- ⅓ cup onion, chopped
- ½ tbsp. Olive oil

To serve:

- 6-7 Whole-wheat taco shells

- 1 cup Purple cabbage, shredded

- Avocado slices

- Chili sauce

- Red pepper flakes

- Cilantro

Directions

1. First, make your marinade by adding all the ingredients to the blender or food processor. Process until smooth and set aside.

2. Create a vertical cut down the center of the pork so it runs from top to bottom. Rub with salt and black pepper. Add oil, onion, and marinade on top, making sure that it gets into the cut part of the pork.

3. Cook on low for about 3 ½ -5 hours (or 2 hours on high). Check after 1 ½ hours and shred pork, put back into the cooker to get more juice in the meat.

4. Once done, set to warm while making the plantains.

5. For the plantains, heat oil in the pan. Add the onions and the plantain. Fry for about 10 minutes.

6. To serve, spoon meat into the taco shells. Add the plantain, avocado, cabbage, red pepper flakes, cilantro, and chili sauce.

Serving: 6-7

Nutritional Facts (per serving): Calories- 212; Carbohydrates- 22.9g; Fats- 6.8g; Protein- 16.3g

Curry Chicken Meatball

Ingredients

For Meatballs:

- 1 pound ground chicken
- tablespoons olive oil
- tsp. Poultry seasoning
- tsp. Dried parsley

For Sauce:

- tbsp. Curry powder
- 1 tsp. Garlic powder
- 1 Large sweet potato, peeled and cubed
- 1/2 cup full-fat coconut cream
- 1 cup Chicken broth
- 13.5 oz. Coconut milk
- 1/2 Medium white onion, chopped
- 1/2 tsp. Salt
- tbsp. Coconut oil

Directions

1   Combine all meatball ingredients in a mixing bowl.

2   Mix thoroughly with your hands.

3   Form meatballs about the size of a ping pong ball.

4   Arrange inside a slow cooker in a single layer.

5   Get another mixing bowl and pour all sauce ingredients over meatballs with the exception of coconut cream.

6   Add sweet potatoes with onions and drizzle it with coconut oil. Cover the lid and cook for 6-8 hours on low or 4 hours on high.

7   Once meatballs are cooked, add full-fat coconut cream and stir to blend.

8   Serve with or over rice as desired.

Servings: 4

Nutritional Facts (per serving): Calories – 623; Carbohydrates – 15g; Fat – 32g; Protein – 224g)

Garlic Chicken with Whole-Wheat Couscous

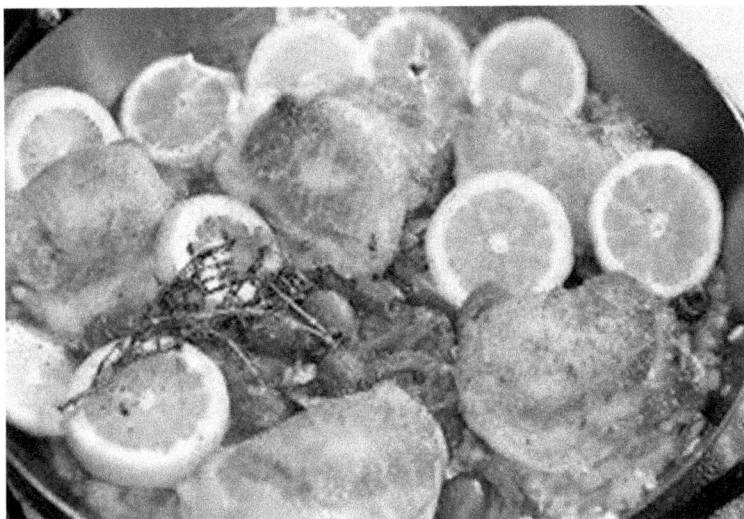

Ingredients

- 1 whole chicken (cut into 6 pieces)

- Coarse salt and ground pepper

- 1 tbsp. Extra-virgin olive oil

- 1 Medium yellow onion, thinly sliced

- Garlic cloves, cut into halves

- tsp. Dried thyme

- 1 cup Dry white wine

- 1/3 cup whole-wheat flour

- 1 cup whole wheat couscous

- Chopped fresh parsley, for serving

Directions

1   Rub chicken with salt and pepper.

2   Preheat a nonstick skillet and add olive oil or coconut oil. Cook the chicken in batches over medium-high heat. Start cooking with chicken's skin down and wait until it turns golden brown in color.

3   Prepare the slow cooker and add onion, thyme, and garlic before layering the chicken pieces on top with skin side up.

4   Cook on high for 3 ½ hours, or if using the low setting on your slow cooker, for 8 hours. Follow properly instruction on the package when cooking whole wheat couscous.

5   Serve chicken over couscous and sprinkle parsley on top.

Serving: 6

Nutritional Facts (per serving): Calories -92; Carbohydrates - 14.55 Fats - 2.86; Protein –2.78

Gluten-Free Salisbury Steak

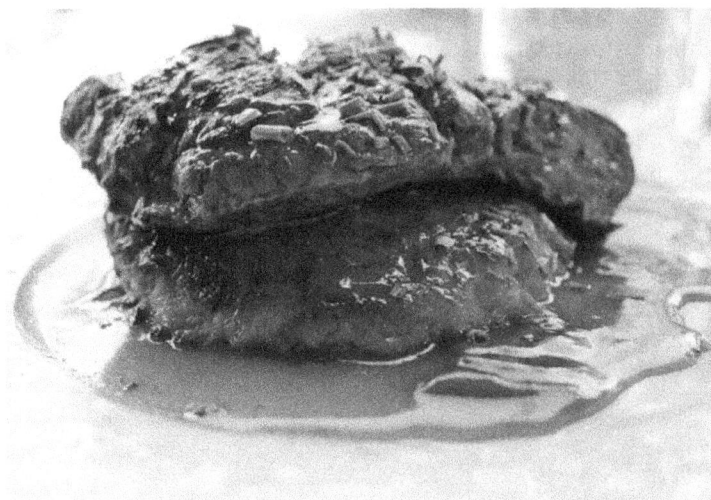

Ingredients

For the steak:

- 2 lb. Grass-fed ground beef

- 1 cup Pork rinds, crushed

- 8 oz. Baby Bella mushrooms

- 2 eggs

- 2 cups Low-sodium beef broth, divided

- 1 cup Onion, chopped

- ¼ cup Ground flaxseed

- ½ tsp. Onion powder

- ½ tsp. Salt

- ¼ tsp. Pepper

For the gravy:

- 1 tsp. Ground dried mustard

- 2 tbsp. Arrowroot powder

- 1 tsp. Worcestershire sauce

- 2 tbsp. Tomato paste

- 1 tbsp. Red wine vinegar

- 1 tsp. Garlic powder

- 1tsp. Olive oil

Directions

1. Put a large skillet over medium heat and sauté the onions until browned.

2. Put the beef, pork rinds, eggs, flaxseed, salt, black pepper, and sautéed onions in a large bowl. Pour in ½ cup of the broth and mix everything well.

3. Make 8 oval-shaped patties and arrange them at the bottom of the crock of the slow cooker. Add the mushrooms on top.

4. Add the gravy ingredients to the remaining broth and mix well. Pour this over the patties and cook on low for 6 hours (or on high for about 3 hours).

Serving: 8

Nutritional Facts: Calories - 486; Carbohydrates - 7.9g; Fats - 26.3g; Protein - 50.7g

Lemongrass Turmeric Slow Cooker Chicken

Ingredients

- 1 can of Lite coconut milk
- 1 lb. of Chicken breast
- 1 stalk of lemongrass
- 1 small shallot
- cloves of garlic
- 1 small red chili (optional)
- tbsp. of fish sauce
- 1 tbsp. of grass-fed butter
- 1 tbsp. of minced fresh ginger
- 1 tbsp. of turmeric powder
- ½ tsp. brown sugar
- Fresh cilantro for garnish
- ½ cup white rice (for serving)

Directions

1   Wash and roughly chop lemongrass, chili, ginger, and shallots. Run them through a food processor and blend with some amount of coconut milk until consistency is smooth.

2   Pour the mixture into the slow cooker and add the fish sauce, sugar, grass-fed butter, and turmeric powder. Also, add the chicken and cover it with the sauce. Cook for 2-3 hours in high.

3   Serve the chicken dish with sauce along with cooked rice and garnish with cilantro.

Serving: 8

Nutritional Facts (per serving): Calories -215; Carbohydrates - 7.64 Fats - 26.91; Protein –26.51

Simple Balsamic Chicken

Ingredients

- 4-6 (about 2.5 lbs.) Boneless, skinless chicken breasts

- ½ cup Balsamic vinegar

- 1 x 16 oz. jar Chunky salsa

Directions

1. Put the chicken breasts to the cooker. Pour the balsamic vinegar and top with salsa and cook the dish on high heat for about 4 hours (or on low for 6 hours).

2. Transfer the chicken breasts to a plate and shred using forks.

3. Put the salsa mixture to a serving bowl. Add the shredded chicken back to the salsa mixture. Serve with lettuce leaves and/or whole wheat bread.

Serving: 6 (serving size of 1 ½ cups)

Nutritional Facts: Calories- 263; Carbohydrates- 8g; Fats- 5g; Protein- 35g

Slow-Cooker Georgia Pulled Pork Barbecue

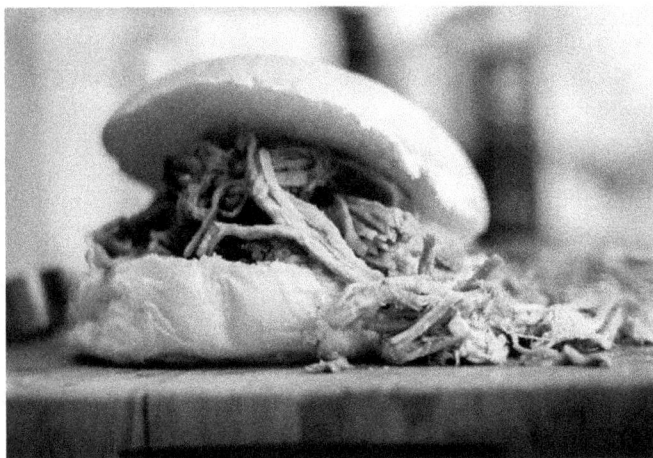

Ingredients

For BBQ Sauce:

- A pinch of cayenne
- 2 cups Cider vinegar
- 1/3 tbsp. Pepper
- 6-oz. Tomato juice
- A dash of hot sauce
- 1 tbsp. Sugar
- 1 tsp. Garlic powder

For Roast

- 4-6 lbs. of pork butt roast, bone-in
- Whole wheat buns for serving
- 1 tsp. Smoked paprika
- 2 tsp. Light Brown sugar
- 2 medium-sized Sweet Onions, quartered
- A pinch of black pepper
- 2 tsp. Salt

Directions

For the Sauce:

1. Put onions in a blender and add ¼ cup of water. Puree until desired consistency.

2. Place pureed onions in a saucepan. Add water to cover and bring to boil. Reduce heat while stirring continuously until the water evaporated almost completely.

3. Add tomato juice, vinegar, hot sauce, cayenne, pepper, and garlic powder. Allow it to simmer before adding in the sugar. Stir and quickly remove from heat. Set a cup of the sauce for the roast while allowing the remaining sauce to cool. Keep inside the fridge for later use.

For the Roast:

1. Spread quartered onions at the bottom of the slow-cooker.

2. In a mixing bowl, combine paprika, salt, and brown sugar and rub this mixture all over the roast. Cook roast in the slow cooker for about 10-12 hours on low heat. Check for tenderness on the 10th hour.

3. Remove roast from the slow cooker and transfer to a platter. Discard the onions.

4. Finely shred meat to pieces. Pour in remaining juice from the slow cooker.

5. Serve on buns.

Serving: 10

Nutritional Facts (per serving): Calories -183; Carbohydrates - 4.1 Fats - 10.77; Protein –31.94

Slow Cooker - Kebabs

Ingredients

- lbs. Chicken meat, cubed

- Fresh green peppers, chopped

- 1 Fresh pineapple, large and cut into chunks

- All-purpose Greek seasoning

- Barbecue sauce

- Pepper

- Salt

- Barbecue skewers

Directions

1   Cleanse chicken in cold water. Also, cleanse the bamboo skewer and set aside for later use. Trim to fit inside your slow cooker.

2   Pat dry the meat in paper towels and season with salt, pepper, and spice blends.

3   Insert the meat, pineapple, and pepper in alternating position into the skewer and arrange inside the slow cooker. Cook on high setting for 4 hours if you don't have much time to wait. You may cook, though on low heat for 8 hours.

4   Remove after allotted time and brush with the BBQ sauce.

5   Grill at high for 1 minute on each side and serve either with salad or other side dishes. This is also best eaten with rice.

Servings: 4

Nutritional Facts (per serving): Calories 379.6; Carbohydrates - 28g; Fat - 7.2g; Protein - 49.5

Slow Cooker Lemon Chicken

Ingredients

- Chicken breasts halves, skinless and bone-in
- 1 tsp. Dried oregano
- 1/2 tsp. Salt
- 1/4 tsp. Pepper
- tbsp. Butter
- 1/4 cup Water
- tbsp. Lemon juice
- Garlic cloves, minced
- tsp. Minced fresh parsley
- Cooked rice

Directions

1   Cleanse the chick and pat dry in paper towels.

2   In a mixing bowl, combine oregano with salt and pepper and rub evenly over chicken breasts.

3   Preheat nonstick skillet over medium heat and brown the butter in olive oil before transferring to the slow cooker.

4   Add water, garlic, and lemon juice extract to the skillet. Bring to boil and loosening bits sticking to the bottom of the skillet. Pour the mixture into the slow cooker. Add the chicken and cover the lid. Cook for about 5-6 hours on low setting.

5   Baste chicken breasts with cooking juices and then add parsley. Cover the dish and continue cooking 15-30 minutes more or until meat juices run clear.

6   Serve with rice.

Note: You may desire to thicken the juice by cooking before serving.

Serving: 6

Nutrition Facts (per serving): Calories – 336; Carbohydrates – 1g; Fat – 10g; Protein – 56g

Slow Cooker Mexican Rice

Ingredients

- 1 cup Chicken stock
- 1 cup White rice
- ½ cup Diced tomatoes in a can
- ½ Jalapeno de-seeded and diced
- ½ tsp. Dried oregano
- ½ tsp. Chili powder
- 1 cup Tomato sauce
- 1 tsp. Cumin
- 4-oz. can Diced green chilies
- ½ tsp. Salt
- ¼ tsp. Pepper
- Fresh Cilantro, to garnish
- Sliced limes, to garnish

Directions

1. Grease inside of slow cooker with olive oil.
2. Add all ingredients with the exception of those for garnishing.
3. Place on the slow cooker the white rice, chicken stock, tomato sauce, diced tomatoes and the rest of the ingredients with the exception of fresh cilantro and limes for garnishing in the slow cooker.
4. Cook on high setting for 2 ½ hours or if on low, set for 5 hours.
5. Garnish with cilantro and lime wedges.

Serving: 4

Nutritional Facts (per serving): Calories -109; Carbohydrates - 19.34 Fats - 1.22g; Protein –3.84g

Slow-Cooker Pineapple Barbecue Sauce Pork Chops

Ingredients

- 6 x 5 oz. Pork Chops

- 1 x 8oz. can Pineapple chunks

- 1 cup Homemade honey barbecue sauce

- 1 Yellow onion, diced

- ⅓ cup Pineapple juice (from the can of pineapple chunks)

- Salt

- Fresh ground pepper

Directions

1. Rub the pork chops with salt and pepper then set aside.

2. Combine the barbecue sauce, pineapple chunks, and onions in a mixing bowl. Mix well.

3. Pour half of the barbecue sauce and the pineapple juice at the bottom of the crock. Arrange the pork chops then pour the remaining sauce mixture over.

4. Cover the cooker with lid and cook on high for about 2 ½- 3 hours (or 4-5 hours on low) until the pork chops are cooked completely.

5. Transfer the pork chops to a serving plate, spooning the sauce over the pork. Best served with brown rice or steamed vegetables.

Serving: 6

Nutritional Facts (per pork chop): Calories- 377; Carbohydrates- 21g; Fats- 15g; Protein- 35g

Slow Cooker Roast Lamb Leg With Gravy

Ingredients

- 4 lb. Lamb leg, bone in (make sure it fits the cooker)

- 2 cups Beef stock

- 2 large garlic cloves, minced

- 1 ½ tsp. Dried thyme

- 1 tbsp. Olive oil

- 1 tsp. Salt

- Black pepper

For the gravy:

- 2 cups Braising liquid from slow cooker, strained

- 3 tbsp. Grass-fed butter

- 3 tbsp. Whole-wheat flour

- Salt

- Pepper

Directions

1. Rub the lamb with salt, pepper, garlic, thyme, and oil on both sides.

2. Pour the beef stock into the cooker and set on low for about 10 hours or until the lamb is tender.

3. Remove from the cooker and transfer to a tray. Lightly drizzle with oil and bake for 20 minutes at 390°F or until browned. Let it rest for 10 minutes before serving.

4. For the gravy, strain the liquid from the cooker using a fine-mesh

465

strainer into a bowl. Measure out 3 cups of liquid, reserving some just in case.

5. Melt the butter in a saucepan over medium heat then add the flour. Cook for about a minute. Add a bit of liquid at a time, whisking as you go. Make sure there are no lumps.

6. Once you poured out all the liquid, adjust heat to medium-high until the gravy thickens. Use the reserved liquid if you need to adjust the consistency.

Serving: 5

Nutritional Facts: Calories- 747; Carbohydrates- 5.2g; Fats- 50.7g; Protein- 63.2g

Spiced Crockpot Beef Roast

Ingredients:

- 1 tsp. Balsamic vinegar
- 2 lbs. of raw boneless beef clod roast
- cloves Garlic, minced
- 1 tbsp. Soy Sauce
- Crockpot spice blend
- cups Whole mushrooms, trimmed
- cups Green beans
- tbsp. Water
- tsp. Worcestershire sauce
- tsp. Dry mustard
- cups of celery stalks, roughly diced
- cups Scallions, chopped
- 1 tbsp. Black pepper
- ½ tsp. Salt

Directions

1. Clear roast of visible fat and cut some slits on top. Rub it black pepper and garlic and put inside the slow cooker.

2. Combine all remaining ingredients except veggies and add to the slow cooker. Cover and cook on slow setting for 8-10 hours or 4-5 hours on high.

3. Add vegetables during the last 30-60 minutes of roasting.

Serving: 4

Nutritional Facts (per serving): Calories -536; Carbohydrates - 7.94 Fats - 28.98; Protein –51.18g

Sweet Potato Chicken

Ingredients

- large carrots, peeled and sliced into rounds

- 1 onion, peeled and sliced

- chicken breasts

- sweet potatoes, peeled and diced

- tbsp. Maple syrup

- tbsp. Olive oil

- Sprigs of fresh thyme

- Salt and pepper to taste

Directions

1   In your slow cooker, add sweet potatoes, carrots, and slices of onions. Pour maple syrup and place the chicken breasts on top seasoned with salt and pepper. Drizzle with olive oil and topped with sprigs of thyme. Set cooker on high for 6 hours and allow it to cook by itself.

Vegan Chana Masala

Ingredients

- 1 tbsp. Olive oil
- 1 tbsp. Freshly grated ginger
- 1 large onion, finely chopped
- garlic cloves, finely minced
- 1/2 tsp. Salt
- 1/4 tsp. Freshly ground pepper
- Thai chilies, diced
- 2 15-oz cans of chickpeas, drained
- 1/2 tsp. Turmeric
- tbsp. Chana Masala seasoning (option: garam masala)
- 3-oz. Tomato paste
- 2 cups Vegetable Broth
- Chopped cilantro, for garnishing
- Cooked rice or naan bread for serving

Directions

1   Heat a little amount of olive oil in a saucepan. Sauté ginger, garlic, and onion – one after the other. Once the onions turn transparent, add peppers, chilies, turmeric, and seasonings. Also, add salt. Cook until chilies become soft and the aroma of the dish lingers.

2   Pour mixture into the slow cooker with tomato paste, vegetable broth, and chickpeas. Cover the slow cooker and cook for 4-6 hours over low heat until sauce thickens. If you desire a thinner sauce, you may add more vegetable broth.

Serving: 4

Nutritional Facts (per serving): Calories -570; Carbohydrates - 66.06 Fats - 17.84g; Protein –38.55g

CONCLUSION

We can't get away from inflammation. It's our body defense against any irritant from outside sources. In a way, any inflammation is a sign that our body immune system is fighting against any undesirable element that is trying to harm us.

However, when inflammation is recurring, it means a more severe underlying cause, hence; we should not neglect any sign of inflammation. To help our body fight against inflammatory elements, it is essential that we take care of what gets into our body, hence; we need to be aware of what we are eating.

Our diet plays an important role in conditioning our body and every food we eat and avoid have their impact on our body functioning and performance.

We had tried our best through this book to give you a better understanding of the significance of the anti-inflammatory diet – particularly on what to eat and what to avoid. This way you can help your body immune system optimize its performance and provide you with better health nourishment.

While most food nutrients, especially in vegetables, are wasted especially in the process of boiling and natural flavors are diminished under high pressure, slow cooker provides a better option for you to minimize if not prevent the escape of valuable nutrients needed by the body.

We have included here delicious and mouth-watering anti-inflammatory recipes which are perfect not only to your taste buds but will likewise help boost your immune system for optimal functioning and performance.

Furthermore, this book provides you with the benefits of a modern kitchen gadget – the slow cooker, thus providing you with the efficacy of preparing a healthy diet for you and your family!

www.ingramcontent.com/pod-product-compliance
Lightning Source LLC
Chambersburg PA
CBHW051708020426

42333CB00014B/889